T0235047

MANAGED CARE

MANAGED CARE

Practice Strategies for Nursing

Margaret M. Conger
with Contributors

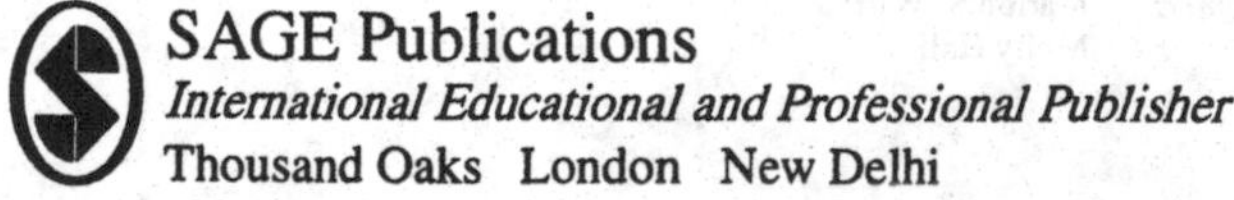

SAGE Publications
International Educational and Professional Publisher
Thousand Oaks London New Delhi

For information:

SAGE Publications, Inc.
2455 Teller Road
Thousand Oaks, California 91320
E-mail: order@sagepub.com

SAGE Publications Ltd.
6 Bonhill Street
London EC2A 4PU
United Kingdom

SAGE Publications India Pvt. Ltd.
M-32 Market
Greater Kailash I
New Delhi 110 048 India

Library of Congress Cataloging-in-Publication Data

Conger, Margaret M.
Managed care: Practice strategies for nursing / by Margaret M. Conger.
p. cm.
Includes bibliographical references and index.
ISBN 0-7619-0964-8 (cloth: acid-free paper)
ISBN 0-7619-0965-6 (pbk.: acid-free paper)
1. Nursing—Effect of managed care on. 2. Nursing—Practice. I. Title.
IN PROCESS
362.1'73'068—dc21 98-40281

98 99 00 01 02 03 04 10 9 8 7 6 5 4 3 2 1

Acquiring Editor: Dan Ruth
Editorial Assistant: Anna Howland
Production Editor: Wendy Westgate
Production Assistant: Nevair Kabakian
Typesetter/Designer: Marion S. Warren
Indexer: Molly Hall

Contents

Preface: "Old Wine in New Wine Skins" **xi**

Acknowledgments xiii

PART I
Managed Care Environment
Preface: Introduction to Managed Care Strategies **1**

1. Health Care Reform: An Opportunity for Nursing **3**
Margaret M. Conger and JoAnne Woodall

The Window of Opportunity 4
Threats to Nursing 5
Managed Health Care Organizations 6
Factors Affecting Health Care Delivery 9
Health Care in the United States 12
Changes Needed in the Health Care System 19
Conclusions 20

2. Managed Care Organizational Structures **23**
Margaret M. Conger

Description of Managed Care 24
Development of Managed Care Organizations 25
Capitation Principles 25

Health Maintenance Organizational Structures 26
Alternate Types of Managed Care Arrangements 30
Elements of Financial Risk 34
For-Profit Versus Not-For-Profit Managed Health Care Plans 36
Federally Financed HMOs 37
Other Federally Financed Health Programs 41
Conclusions 43

3. Managed Care Organizational Strategies Used to Achieve Organizational Goals **47**
Margaret M. Conger

Integration of Services 48
Coordination of Care 51
Health Promotion Strategies 57
Quality Management 61
Conclusions 64

4. Nursing Involvement in Quality of Care Issues **67**
Margaret M. Conger

Traditional Quality Measurement Techniques 68
Specific Quality Indicators 74
Ethical Principles 80
Model for Assessing the Quality of Nursing Care 82
Measurement of Cost-Effectiveness 83
Conclusions 87

5. Nursing Case Management: A Managed Care Organizational Strategy **91**
Margaret M. Conger

Origins of Nursing Case Management 92
Definitions of Nursing Case Management 94
Models of Nurse Case Management 95
Goals of Nurse Case Management 97
Skills Required for Nurse Case Management 99
Who Is the Case Manager? 101
Educational Preparation for Nurse Case Management 102
Which Clients Require Case Management? 105
Conclusions 107

PART II
Nursing Strategies in Acute-Care Hospitals **111**

6. Use of Nurse Extenders **113**
Margaret M. Conger

Reasons for Use of Nurse Extenders 114
Who Is the Nurse Extender? 115
Educational Programs for Unlicensed Nurse Personnel 119
What Is the Role of the RN When Working With the UAP? 120
Education Needed for Registered Nurses for Effective Teamwork 123
Clinical Example 129
Conclusions 132

7. Advanced Practice Nurses: Acute-Care Settings **135**
Margaret M. Conger

Advanced Practice Nurse Roles in Acute-Care Settings 136
Acute-Care Nurse Practitioner 142
Overlap Between CNS and ACNP Roles 147
Conclusions 149

8. Nurse Case Management: Acute-Care Hospital Practice **153**
Margaret M. Conger and JoAnne Woodall

Admission Activities 154
Concurrent Review 159
Functions of the Nurse Case Manager During the Hospital Stay 167
Discharge Process 171
Conclusions 173

9. Automated Clinical Pathways in the Patient Record: Legal Implications **175**
Lisa Brugh

The Clinical Pathway 176
The Clinical Pathway as a Documentation Tool 177
Interdisciplinary Clinical Pathway Development 179

Outcome-Focused Care 181
Example of an Automated Clinical Pathway 182
Legal Implications 185
Legal Considerations for Use of Computer Documentation System 190
Conclusions 191

10. Clinical Pathway Outcome Research **195**
Pamela Keberlein

Examples of Outcome Studies 196
Research Study 197
Conclusions 204

PART III
Nursing Strategies in Community Settings **207**

11. Nurse Case Management in Community Settings **209**
Margaret M. Conger

Long-Term Care 210
Home-Based Programs 212
Parish Nursing 215
Physician Office Case Management 219
Conclusions 221

12. Population-Based Nurse Case Management **223**
Margaret M. Conger

Population-Based Case Management 224
Methods Used in Population-Based Case Management 224
Case Management Based on Living Circumstances 226
Case Management of Special-Needs Infants 228
Case Management of High-Risk Pregnancy 230
Case Management of the Elderly 230
Conclusions 236

13. Advanced Practice Nurses as Case Managers **239**
Margaret M. Conger and Carol E. Craig

Advanced Practice Role: Nurse Case Manager 240

Disease-Specific Nurse Case Management 243
Conclusions 254

14. Advanced Practice Roles in Community Settings: Community Health Clinics **257**
Carol E. Craig, Kathy Ingleses, and Margaret M. Conger

Health Management: The Teen Population 258
Health Management: Uninsured Populations 262
Conclusions 265

15. Advanced Nurse Collaborative Practice in a Primary Care Setting **269**
Carol E. Craig and Margaret M. Conger

Need for APNs in Primary Health Care Settings 270
Evolving Roles for Advanced Practice Nurses 271
Model of Collaborative Practice Between APNs 271
Example From Clinical Practice 273
Advanced Practice Roles for Nurses in the Center 274
Uniqueness of APN Collaboration 276
Evaluation Methodologies 278
Client Situations 279
Conclusions 281

Index **283**

About the Editor **288**

About the Contributors **289**

Preface: "Old Wine in New Wine Skins"

We have long been told that new wine in old wineskins will cause the skins to burst (Matthew 9:17). Perhaps today we need to turn this around and think about the effect of old wine in new wineskins. Many nurses are still trying to shape their practice to methods that have worked in the past—but health care delivery systems have changed. What is needed now is to invent new ways to deliver nursing care in the new environment. The purpose of this book is to provide nurses with an opportunity to explore the new environment (the wine skin) and how to produce new wine—nursing practices that meet the new health care environment's needs. The changes that managed health care is bringing will be explored; ways that nurses can grow professionally in this new environment will then be discussed.

Nursing students need to understand the changing world of health care that they will encounter on entry into practice. Staff nurses also need to have a resource to assist them in understanding the changes they encounter on a daily basis. It is hoped that this book will assist both neophyte nurses and those who have long been established in practice to take steps to manage the destiny of nursing.

Many of the elements important to nursing in the past are still relevant to practice today, but these elements need to be recast to meet the needs of the new environment. Old recipes for winemaking need not be discarded, just adapted to the present environment. With the current market pressures moving health care toward an emphasis of wellness promotion, avoidance of illness, and efficient management of expensive resources, nurses are in an excellent position to move into this new paradigm. Long-held nursing ideals such as focusing on health and wellness, patient advocacy, and caring for the individual within the context of his or her environment are vital to successful practice in the changing environment. It is a paradox that our future survival will, in part, be determined by our ability to return to some of our fundamental roots. Florence Nightingale left an indelible stamp on the nursing profession when over a century ago she advocated for nurses to

> care for the sick at home as well as in the hospital, and to serve all kinds and classes of people, rich and poor, the mentally disabled, and families and communities as well as individuals. The teaching of health maintenance and the prevention of sickness is to be an important part of their work. (Hay, 1993, p. 149)

These principles are still relevant today. Managed care organizations are beginning to place economic value on health promotion rather than on a singular focus on the technical care of acute health crises. This new concern for health promotion is an opportunity that nursing must not miss. Now is the time to reinvent nursing to meet the challenges of the managed care environment.

This book is about the managed care health system and the changes that it has brought to nursing. The managed care movement will be examined in the first section of this book. The foundational principles upon which it operates will be explored and the terminology used to describe the multitude of forms that it can take will be introduced. A brief review of the history of medical care in the past 50 years will also be discussed to provide a basis for understanding why change was necessary. The concerns that nurses are expressing about their future will also be examined.

After a foundation has been laid for understanding the important elements of managed care, the remainder of the book will focus on strategies that are being used by nurses to conduct their practice in the emerging health care system. Many of the strategies discussed are useful both in the more familiar acute-care hospital-based practice and in the multitude of newly emerging community settings. Nurses, armed with both learning from past experience and knowledge about the pressures, needs, and trends of the current health care marketplace, will be in a strong position to mold and shape their own future.

Acknowledgments

This book is a reflection of the thinking of many people. First and foremost, much of the content has grown out of conversations between JoAnne Woodall and myself as we spent a year driving once a week from Flagstaff to Tucson, Arizona to study case management at the University of Arizona. I am also grateful for the wisdom, insight, and leadership of Rose Gerber, RN, PhD, of the University of Arizona for allowing JoAnne and me to study nursing case management along with the University of Arizona graduate students. Finally, much of the content of this book has been reviewed, discussed, and even challenged by my graduate students at Northern Arizona University. All of these people have had a significant impact on the content included in this book. Without the input and encouragement of each of these people, this project would not have been possible.

MARGARET M. CONGER
NORTHERN ARIZONA UNIVERSITY

Reference

Hay, M. (1993, October). Nursing's renaissance. *Health Progress, 74*(3), 26-32.

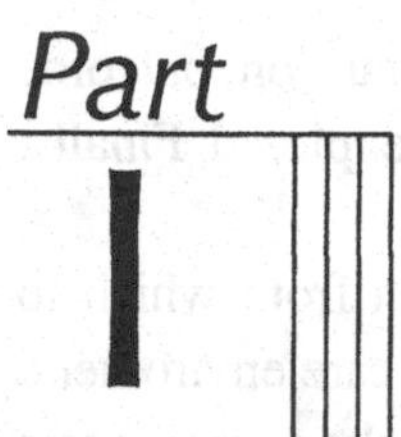

Part I

Managed Care Environment

Preface: Introduction to Managed Care Strategies

Changes in health care delivery systems in recent years have had a profound effect on how providers of care function. These changes have caused great upheaval in practice patterns, but they can also be an opportunity for growth for the nursing profession. However, growth cannot occur unless nurses understand the functioning of managed care systems and learn to use the values of such systems in altering nursing care practices. In this section of the book, managed care strategies will be explored and terminology used to describe the new system will be explained.

The first chapter will explore the history of health care in the United States during the last 50 years, establishing a basis for understanding why change is necessary. The reader will then be introduced to the various structures used in managed health care organization to achieve the goals of cost-effectiveness, quality care, and access to care. The three chapters dealing with these topics will serve as an introduction to managed care principles.

The last two chapters of this section will focus more specifically on nursing practices that affect both quality of care and cost-effective care.

Measurement of quality of care, with a particular focus on outcome measurements that relate directly to nursing care, will be explored. Finally, the use of nurses as case managers will be introduced.

The first section of this book provides a foundation from which to understand specific nursing strategies used in a managed care enviroment. With this knowledge, the nurse will be well positioned to take an active role in shaping health care delivery systems that will meet the needs of the public in these times of rapid changes.

Chapter

1 Health Care Reform

An Opportunity for Nursing

Margaret M. Conger
JoAnne Woodall

"We can never go back to before."
—*Ragtime* (musical by T. McNally)

Health care delivery in the United States is undergoing profound change. What has been in the past is gone and will probably never return. Instead, health care providers need to learn new ways to succeed in the changing environment. This new health care system is referred to as *managed care*, words that bring fear to many, both providers as well as recipients of health care. However, fear can be conquered through knowledge. It is essential that health care professionals become informed about the values inherent in the managed care system and the strategies used in its operation. Nurses, in particular, who make up a substantial portion of health care providers, need to become knowledgeable about these changes. Rather than remaining on the sidelines as observers, they must become active in shaping the development of the managed care environment. The emerging health care environment must be viewed as a window of opportunity for positive change rather than as a threat.

The Window of Opportunity

Any period of upheaval can be viewed as an opportunity for growth or as a period of disorganization or crisis. Nurses must analyze what this changing environment means, both in the present and for the future. Does this change represent a threat to the future, or is it an opportunity for positive change or growth for the nurse as a professional? The alternatives must be considered because in the emerging health care environment, as in any changing system, it is the leaders, not the followers, who will survive and succeed (Sovie, 1995). Curtin (1994) suggests that this is the time for nursing to reinvent itself.

Nurses need to take charge of their own destiny and find their place in the new health care system. It is up to them to help create and cement the culture in which nursing values will be stressed. This cannot be done by simply adjusting to the changes going on in the health care environment; it must be done by leading the change. New nursing roles are needed for this process. The role of the advanced practice nurse is integral to this redefinition. An emerging role for the advanced practice nurse is that of the nurse case manager. Other roles, such as the nurse practitioner, nurse midwife, and nurse anesthetist, are also needed for the new environment. All of these will be vital to reaching the goals of managed care organizations.

Also, it is not productive for nurses to simply protest the changes. Instead of being devalued by the managed care system, nurses need to demonstrate added value in decreasing health care costs, improving health outcomes, and promoting consumer satisfaction. In doing so, nurses will not only insure the survival of their profession; they will emerge stronger by becoming essential to the survival of the health care system.

The entire change process is a learning adventure. Mezirow (1994) identifies important elements of learning that take place when adults critically examine a significant event. This learning is reflected by nurses as they experience the process of change in response to and in anticipation of their changing environment. Mezirow suggests that learning can be initiated as the result of exposure to a disorienting dilemma. The health care evolution could certainly be described as a dilemma for nurses, the impact of which is confusion, disorientation, and insecurity. Mezirow further suggests that following recognition of a dilemma, a person is more open to exploring the possibility of developing new roles, relationships, and actions. This phase of learning is the window of opportunity for nurses in redefining their roles and creating new ones to meet the challenges and expectations. Mezirow further suggests that in a time of such change, a new course of action must be planned, and the new skills and knowledge needed for implementation of the plan must be developed. The new roles must be tried out and relationships must be renegotiated. Developing a new role for nursing is, then, the response that is needed for the changes in the health care system. This is an opportunity that nurses must seize.

Threats to Nursing

The changes in the health care system can provide an opportunity for nursing, but there are also a number of threats present. Many hospital administrators, faced with the challenges produced by this new environment, are taking a hard look at their expenditures. They are looking at reducing staffing costs, which often represent 50% or more of the total cost per patient. Nurses are rightly concerned about this trend because they make up a large proportion of hospital staff. Of nurses presently in active practice, two thirds are employed by hospitals (Coile, 1995). The quick fix, as seen by many administrators, is to reduce the number of nurses providing hospital care. It is not surprising, then, that many nurses see the future in terms of job threats, reduced pay, and reduced opportunity. This bleak outlook for nurses is reinforced by Coile, who suggests that nursing will not be able to control its own destiny: rather, economic forces will be in control of nursing's future.

In the wake of the current health care changes, nursing is facing possible obsolescence. The financial pressures faced by hospitals are being transmitted to nurses in the form of lower wages, fewer opportunities for advancement, lesser wage differentials for professional education and training, and increased layoffs. In addition, staffing patterns using non-R.N. substitutes for the registered nurse are becoming common. The picture can be grim, with the prospect of a surplus of nurses leading to decreased value such as occurs when supply exceeds demand. Compounding this downward spiral is the prospect of nurses being placed in the middle of ethical dilemmas when cost-cutting pressures leading to early discharge of patients conflict with nurses' commitment to patient advocacy and quality care. The picture that emerges is that of nursing caught up and tossed about by change. As nurses take stock of the damages that have resulted from changes in the workplace, they find they are working harder for less wages and diminished satisfaction.

This, then, is the challenge facing nursing in this time of radical change. Nurses must be involved in the reinvention of nursing. The new skills and relationships required for success in the emerging health care environment must be mastered—and even as new roles are emerging, the entire situation must continually be reassessed. This is not the time for complacency. It has been said that nothing is certain but change itself. The hope and expectation is that, as nurses successfully negotiate their new role in the health care system, they will become more expert in learning from the past, in reading current trends to understand the present, and in making educated predictions about the future. By doing so, they will be favorably positioned to create change rather than just to react to it. Their role in the emerging health care system will be enhanced rather than diminished. To be successful in this process, a well-founded understanding of the managed care environment is necessary.

Managed Health Care Organizations

Managed health care organizations have arisen in the United States to provide a new approach to the health delivery system. Their goal is to provide a comprehensive range of services to an enrolled population at a fixed premium. The aim of a well-run organization is to deliver high-quality medical care at a competitive price. To be successful, these organizations have had to find ways to meet the health needs of enrolled members with a limited amount of revenue (MacLeod, 1995).

The movement into managed care has occurred rapidly. Ten years ago, most Americans could not even describe a managed health care organization. However, in the November 1996 bulletin of the American Association of Retired People, it was reported that more than half of all Americans are now enrolled in a managed care organization. Also, 10% of all Medicare beneficiaries have opted for this type of care rather than the fee-for-service care that has been their traditional option (Coppola, Croft, & Leo, 1997). This rapid change to managed care has not been easy and has left many people in doubt about what it means to their own health care. Also, questions about how to provide quality health care in the face of such rapid change have arisen.

Common concerns include issues about consumer protection and balancing cost effectiveness with quality.

In the rapidly emerging environment of managed care and integrated health systems, hospitals and other provider institutions are reeling from the effects of the rapid economic changes. These institutions are being forced to make drastic changes in philosophy and function to remain relevant and viable (Himali, 1995). Instead of profiting when their expensive, highly technical services are heavily used, as in the past, they are now forced to look at the realities of payment systems in which rewards are achieved by keeping people out of the expensive treatment systems. Treatment in the most resource-efficient environment is now the goal (Turner, 1995). This reality is requiring hospitals and other provider institutions to look at downsizing, reducing expenditures, and keeping people healthy.

A paradigm shift has occurred. In the old system, profit was made from treating illness; in the new system, survival depends on keeping people well and treating them with a conservative eye on the bottom line (Sovie, 1995). Profit can no longer be made with high expenditures for the relatively few high-risk, high-acuity, high-cost patients. In the new paradigm, survival is dependent on increasing the volume of low-risk patients requiring a lesser level of service. As a result, providers are battling for these low health need patients, resulting in a highly competitive market. To compete in this marketplace, providers must look not only at reducing costs and increasing volume; they must also demonstrate quality performance, gaining high marks on their "report card" for positive clinical outcomes and patient satisfaction.

Common Characteristics

Although managed care has a variety of permutations, it can be understood generally as a health system that is designed and implemented to organize and manage the delivery of services in such a way that limited resources are controlled (Hinitz-Satterfield, Miller, & Hagan, 1993).

There are several strategies used by most managed care organizations in an attempt to lower health care costs. These are shown in Table 1.1. One is to restrict members of the organization to using predetermined services that are provided at discounted fees. Enrollees are required to use predetermined doctors and hospitals that have agreed to provide care at discounted rates. If

TABLE 1.1 Strategies Common to Managed Care Organizations

- Restrict member use to predetermined services and providers
- Use of gatekeepers to control access to services
- Use of prior approval for use of
  - Testing
  - Treatments
  - Speciality care
- Increased availability of health promotion activities
- Increased health education opportunities
- Increased delivery of care within the community
  - Day surgeries
  - Outpatient laboratory testing
  - Outpatient diagnostic services
  - Increased use of subacute-care settings
  - Increased use of home health services

a member chooses to go outside of the approved list of providers, he will be required to either pay for all of the cost of care or, at best, pay the difference between the amount charged by the approved provider and the outside provider.

There also are restrictions on how the person will access the system. The use of a "gatekeeper," in which a primary care provider oversees the care of the enrollee and determines when the resources of a specialist are needed, is prevalent. All requests for treatment are funneled through this person. The gatekeeper is also held responsible for coordinating care so that duplication of services is eliminated.

To maintain cost effectiveness, there is also an emphasis on avoiding overuse of testing, treatments, and speciality care. One way this is done is to require prior approval from the managed care organization for all medical procedures. The health care organization will also control when a member is allowed to use the services of the hospital, home health care agency, or other outpatient services. Consequently, the health care consumer will find fewer choices when choosing a physician, hospital, or other health agency and, many times, even the services that will be provided.

Another strategy used by managed care organizations is to increase opportunities for members to participate in health promotion activities. The emphasis has shifted from a primary concern with illness management common in the traditional fee-for-service structure to services designed to assist enrolled members in remaining healthy. Thus health education programs have proliferated. Preventive measures, such as immunizations and screening programs, are also an important part of the managed care organization strategy.

Another significant change brought about by the managed care environment is the movement to provide an emphasis on care based in the community. This has resulted in increased use of outpatient services such as day surgeries, laboratory testing, and diagnostic services (Venegoni, 1996). It has also led to significant increases in the development of subacute-care settings such as rehabilitative long-term care agencies and nursing homes. This movement into the community has led to an enormous increase in the growth of the home health industry, which is reported to be the fastest growing segment of health care (Olsten Health, 1997). All in all, the managed care movement is radically changing the way health care is delivered in the United States.

Factors Affecting Health Care Delivery

A number of factors in the marketplace have had a profound effect on the changes occurring in the health care industry. The rise in health care costs in the United States in the past two decades, which has exceeded the rate of inflation, has been a strong impetus to bring about change. The per capita health care expenditure increased from $400 in 1970 to $2,400 in 1989. It was estimated that in 1996, one seventh of the economy of the United States would be spent on health care (Abbey, 1997). Also, the percentage of health care costs paid by the consumer rather than a third-party payer have risen considerably. The average monthly premium paid by the worker for family health coverage has increased from $45 in 1983 to $107 in 1993. This is on top of much higher deductible amounts that the consumer is also paying (*Seattle Times*, 1996). With health care costs escalating at this rapid rate, there is pressure from many sources to control further cost increases. Market forces have been a major influence on changing the way health care delivery is provided. The relationship of the market forces at work to bring health care costs under control is depicted in Figure 1.1. Employers who have paid for a large share of health care costs have spurred the movement by shopping for better prices and looking for better health outcomes for their money (Ermann, 1988). They are looking for both effectiveness of care and efficiency in providing the care (Riley, 1994). At the same time, providers have been faced

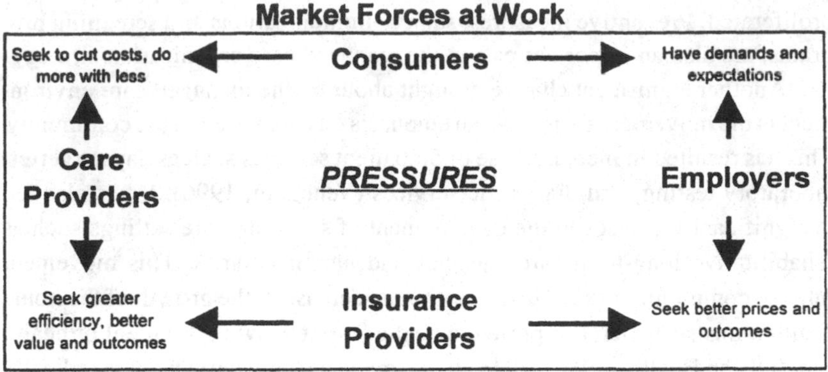

Figure 1.1 Effect of Market Forces on the Health Care System

with cutting costs to remain competitive for contracts with insurance companies. New ways to provide cost-effective care that meets the demands of the consumers had to be found. To complicate the picture further, consumer expectations for state-of-the-art health care continue to rise. With such a multiplicity of variables, it is little wonder that profound changes are occurring in the health care delivery system in this country.

Many problems are associated with the rapid change to managed care. Perhaps the most significant problem is that of learning to balance cost effectiveness with quality. Because the change is occurring so rapidly, quality standards have not been established. To illustrate the importance placed on this issue, in the fall of 1996, President Clinton announced the formation of a Presidential Advisory Commission on Consumer Protection and Quality. The charge given to this commission was to make recommendations on how best to ensure the quality of health care and patient protection.

Other organizations have also addressed this issue. One such agency is the National Committee on Quality Assurance (NCQA), a private nonprofit agency that has developed 50 standards by which to evaluate the operations of a managed care organization. Because this is a voluntary process, not every managed care organization has been evaluated using these standards. However, as of September 1996, about 300 managed care organizations had been reviewed (American Association of Retired Persons Special Bulletin, 1996).

Of these, 101 plans received a full 3-year accreditation, 85 plans received 1-year accreditation with specific improvement plans, 26 received provisional accreditation, and 24 were denied accreditation. It is expected that this type of accreditation will increase.

Hospitals that are associated with managed care organizations will continue to seek accreditation in more traditional ways, such as through the Joint Commission on the Accreditation of Health Care Organizations (JCAHO). In addition, the Health Care Financing Administration (HCFA), which oversees the Medicare health care system, is also carrying out reviews of managed care organizations that have special plans targeted to the elderly population. HCFA is looking at such issues as appropriateness and cost of treatment, possible premature discharges, outcomes of treatment, and consumer satisfaction (Ermann, 1988).

In addition to these more formal organizations, a number of consumer-oriented quality review groups have arisen. The Consumer Coalition for Quality Health Care is such a group. It has developed an instrument called a Quality Compass for use in collecting information from managed care plans. Reports on scores achieved by managed care organizations are available by request from the organization. Another private consumer group is the Coalition for Health Care Choice and Accountability. This coalition is calling for national standards by which to judge the effectiveness of managed care organizations. *U.S. News and World Report*, the American Association of Retired Persons (AARP), and the Consumers Union have also evaluated managed care plans. It is expected that, with this increase in evaluation of managed care organizations, more interest in means to achieve quality health care outcomes as well as cost outcomes will develop. This would be an important step in providing for consumer protection in the health care environment.

Along with consumer groups that are searching for effective means to evaluate managed care organizations, a number of states have also developed legislation by which to better regulate managed care organizations. Recent legislation in several states mandated second-day stays following childbirth if recommended by a physician. This movement has also spread to the federal level, and now such stays are mandated in all states. Unfortunately, this type of control is very "piecemeal" and could lead to very fragmented quality control, as well as increased costs whose need has not been demonstrated. It seems that a more global approach to quality issues would be a better way to protect consumer interests.

Health Care in the United States

Health care in the United States has undergone considerable change during the period following World War II. What has caused these changes in care delivery? And what are the driving forces causing the current upheaval in health care? To fully understand the current health care environment, one must first step back and look at where health care has been.

Boom Times: 1950 to 1980

The period between 1950 and 1980 is often referred to as a "boom time" for health care.

A number of factors shown in Figure 1.2 shaped the health care industry during the post–World War II period. The economy in the United States was rapidly growing, with no fears for the future. There was little competition from foreign markets. Remember when "Made in Japan" was considered the stamp of a shoddy product? This was also a period when the population as a whole felt responsible for the social ills of the country; it was the era of Johnson's "Great Society." At this time, health care was considered by both the government and business to be a right for each person (Bernstein, 1996; Langston, 1992).

Response to these values was a rapid increase in employer- and government-sponsored health care plans that served to distance the consumer of health care from the cost of health care. Because health care expenditures were not paid for directly by the consumer, the individual person paid little attention to either cost or overuse. The employers also showed little concern about rising health care costs because their business profits were continually rising and thus the yearly increases for health care were affordable (Anderson, 1989).

Another factor in increasing the cost of health care came from the introduction of health care plans sponsored by the federal government. Medicare legislation (Title XVIII, Social Security Act) passed in 1965 provided health insurance for people 65 and older. Prior to this legislation, this group had very limited health care choices because they did not benefit from the rapid expansion of employer-sponsored health care plans. The provision of health care payments for the elderly greatly increased the demand for services (Bernstein, 1996). The Medicaid program (Title XIX, Social Security Act),

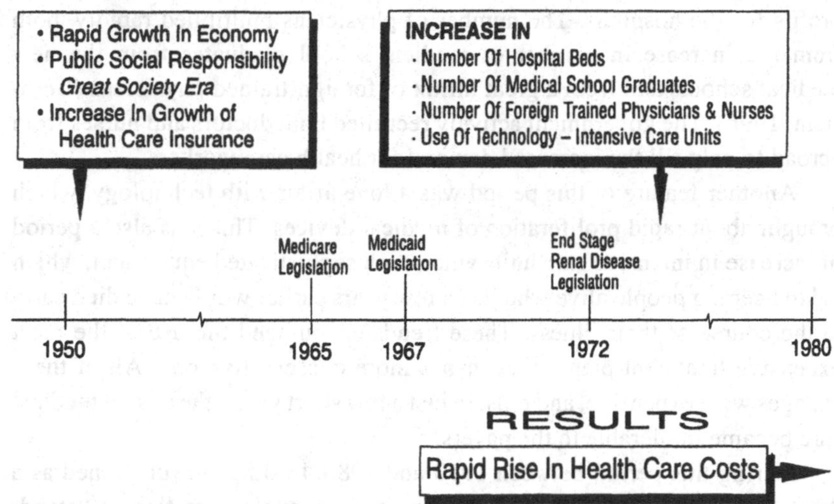

Figure 1.2 Boom Times in Health Care

passed in 1967, provided health care coverage for the medically uninsured poor. This further increased the number of people now eligible for health care. Bernstein (1996) suggests that this provision of health care coverage for the elderly and the poor was one of the most significant legislative achievements of the Kennedy-Johnson era.

The role of the government in providing funding for health care in the United States was further expanded in 1972 with legislation to include people with end-stage renal disease (ESRD) under the Medicare program. The health costs that resulted from this legislation have been far greater than ever anticipated. The number of people living with ESRD in 1973 at the initiation of the program was around 10,000 (Rettig, 1996). By 1997, the number of Americans living with ESRD was over 300,000—a 30-fold increase (Stevens, 1997). The management of a person with ESRD is a very expensive service, at an estimated cost per person per year of $36,000. The mean number of years for a person to remain on dialysis is about 15 (Friedman, 1996).

To provide for the increased demand for health care by Medicare and Medicaid beneficiaries, the number of hospitals and health care workers increased dramatically (Bernstein, 1996). The Hill-Burton Act provided funding for building of hospitals and medical schools. With the increase in health insurance funding, the new hospital beds remained full and led to even bigger profits for the hospitals. The number of physicians multiplied rapidly, both from the increase in number of medical school graduates from the new medical schools and from a great influx of foreign-trained physicians (Bernstein, 1996). The government actively recruited both doctors and nurses from abroad to help fill the increased demand for health care workers.

Another feature of this period was a love affair with technology, which brought about rapid proliferation of medical devices. This was also a period of increase in intensive care units with much sophisticated equipment, which led to keeping people alive who just a few years earlier would have died early in the course of their illness. These trends encouraged the use of the most expensive treatment plan rather than a more conservative one. All of these changes were expensive, and thus, in just a few short years, the cost of medical care became intolerable to the payers.

During this period between 1950 and 1980, health care functioned as a "cottage industry," with both physicians and hospitals operating in "stand-alone" arrangements. There was little movement to integrate services into larger organizations. Providers—both physicians and hospitals—were in competition for the consumers of health services. Each hospital attempted to get the most sophisticated equipment available and offer every medical service in an attempt to attract both physicians and their patients to use their facility. This resulted in tremendous duplication of services in a community. Regulation of the health care industry was very limited, and little attempt was made to curtail duplication of services among competing hospitals. Again, these practices led to significant increases in health care costs.

Hospitals were evaluated by a voluntary accreditation program through the Joint Commission for Accreditation of Hospitals (JCHO), now known as the Joint Commission on Accreditation of Health Care Organizations (JCAHO). At this time, the focus of accreditation was on the structures in place used to document the credentials of the physician and nursing staff. Emphasis was also placed on reviewing policy and procedure manuals to determine processes used. Finally, the state of the physical plant was considered very important. Patient outcomes resulting from the care provided were not evaluated.

The result of all of these factors present from 1950 to 1980 resulted in uncontrolled growth of the health care industry. Health care costs in the United States were rising far more rapidly than other segments of the economy. It was critically important to alter health care practices to bring some type of order out of the chaos created during this period.

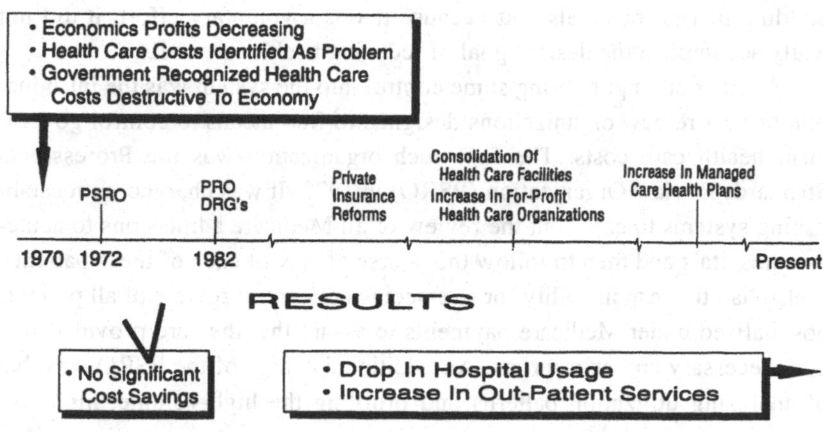

Figure 1.3 Hard Reality

Hard Reality: 1980 to the Present

By the early 1980s, the world economic picture had begun to change, with the realization that health care costs had to be contained if economic survival was to be achieved (Anderson, 1989). A number of factors converged to force a change in the way health care delivery would be provided. These changes are outlined in Figure 1.3.

Many manufacturing companies found that they could not compete in the global economy because products could be made more cheaply in developing countries than in the United States. The portion of the manufacturing budget allocated to labor costs was of great concern. Looking at manufacturing costs, it is readily apparent that health care costs were one of the major contributors to the escalating cost of doing business. Thus, businesses began to look at ways to reduce this cost. The federal government also recognized that the increase in health care costs could not continue without destroying the economy of the country. In this way, then, the two major payers for the health care industry actively began to seek solutions to control health care expenditures (Anderson, 1989).

One attempt to control health care costs was to develop regional planning groups to better control the building of hospital beds and the acquisition of new equipment (Anderson, 1989). This attempt did slow somewhat the building of new hospitals, but because it was a voluntary effort, it did not really accomplish the desired goal of reducing health care costs.

Another attempt to bring some control into the system was the introduction of peer review organizations designed to find means to control government health care costs. The first such organization was the Professional Standards Review Organization (PSRO) in 1972. It was charged with establishing systems to carry out the review of all Medicare admissions to acute-care hospitals and then to follow the course of stay of each of these patients. It also had the responsibility for overseeing concurrent review of all patients hospitalized under Medicare payments to assure that the care provided was both necessary and appropriate. An additional charge of the PSRO was that of analyzing utilization patterns and profiling the high-volume, high-cost admissions.

Because the activities of the PSRO were primarily a retrospective review of health care provided, there was little effect on curbing health care expenditures. No statistical significance was found to support the idea that the PSRO review altered the length of stay or days of care per 1000 Medicare enrollees. There was some evidence to support the belief that the PSRO activity led to an increase in quality of care. When the work of the PSRO was reviewed, it was concluded that the cost of carrying out the program equaled any saving found in delivering health care (Ermann, 1988).

In 1982, the PSRO was supplanted by a new group, the Peer Review Organization (PRO), which is still in existence today. The goals developed for this organization were to ensure that health care services provided were medically necessary, provided in an appropriate setting, and met recognized standards for quality. The charge given to the PRO was to review 25% of all Medicare admissions; do preadmission screening for need for acute hospital care; do presurgery screening, requiring the use of a second opinion prior to surgery; and carry out concurrent review of all Medicare patients in acute-care hospitals. Part of this program was the use of denial of payment to a hospital if it could be determined that an admission was not medically necessary (Ermann, 1988).

Data gathered by the Health Care Financing Administration (HCFA) indicate that the PRO reviews have been somewhat successful in reducing health care costs. Data for 1985 showed that PRO groups screened 46% of all Medicare admissions to acute-care hospitals. In postdischarge review of patient charts, 2.67% of all admissions were found inappropriate and thus payment for the care was denied to the hospital. It was estimated that the PRO had saved the government $176 million. This resulted in a cost/benefit ratio of 1:1.2; that is, for every dollar spent, $1.20 was saved (Ermann, 1988).

Another attempt on the part of the United States government to control health care costs of the elderly was the introduction of the Diagnostic Related Groups (DRG) in 1982. In this system, a fixed amount of money was allocated to cover the costs of health care for a specific medical diagnosis during an acute-care hospitalization (Long, 1994). The amount of money provided was based on an intensive study done in New Jersey to determine the average cost of care for a particular diagnosis such as a myocardial infarction. Rather than using a retrospective payment system in which the government paid whatever bills were submitted for a Medicare beneficiary's care, the hospital received a fixed, prospectively determined amount of money. If the care could be provided for less than the amount of money stipulated, the hospital could keep the excess. However, if the care cost more than the stipulated amount, the hospital took the excess cost as a loss. Also, if the patient was readmitted to the hospital soon after discharge with the same diagnosis, it was considered as the same admission and no additional funding was provided. This policy was established to prevent the hospital from prematurely discharging patients and then readmitting them for further care. Private insurance companies quickly followed the example of the government and also put limits on the amount of money paid for specific diagnoses. The response to the introduction of the DRG system was a very rapid decrease in hospital usage and an increase in outpatient delivery of health care.

The decreased length of stay in the acute-care hospital has been a major factor in fueling the phenomenal increase in home health services. The Federal Bureau of Labor Statistics projects that there will be an increase of more than 500,000 jobs in the home health industry between 1992 and 2005 (Olsten Health, 1997). This works out to be a 128% increase in job opportunities. Similar changes in delivery of services, such as outpatient surgery and outpatient diagnostic services, have also occurred (Venegoni, 1996).

The private health insurance plans also responded to the ever rising health care costs and made attempts to control these expenditures. They began to increase the out-of-pocket expenses for employees, thus giving the individual a better sense of the cost of health care. This was done in the form of larger copayments required of the enrolled members. A movement also began that would limit the number of health care choices for the employee. Private insurance plans contracted with specific health care providers to provide care at a "discount" for enrolled members. They were able to negotiate these contracts because the provider would realize a larger volume of patients as the result of this exclusive contract. If a person chose to go to a physician or hospital not within the contract, that employee would pay the difference in price between the contracted service and the chosen service (Wagner, 1997).

During this period there was a rapid rise in consolidations and mergers of health care organizations and systems. It was found that by increasing the size of the organization, costs could be reduced. For example, organizations that could buy products in volume were able to negotiate a lower price (Menke, 1997). Also, by integrating services, costs could be reduced by providing the more expensive services at fewer locations. Thus, the cottage industry phases of health care began to disappear.

Another phenomenon of this period was the dramatic increase in "for-profit" health care systems. These systems were able to raise large amounts of capital and buy out many of the small hospitals built under the Hill-Burton Act. The for-profit economic motive has tended to focus more on the return of profit to the shareholder than on the public good of the community or "social capital." As the number of private, community-based hospitals began to diminish, the traditional value of providing health care to all despite the ability to pay also began to disappear (Coppola et al., 1997). It is estimated that by 1994, 40 million Americans had no health care coverage (Weissman, 1996). This represents about 17% of the population. This number is probably on the increase with the changing demographics of employment. Thus, one must question what the effect of a system that is based on the profit motive rather than the good of the community will be on the health of the country.

All of these issues are important to the rise of managed care health plans. The switch from a retrospective, cost-based reimbursement system to a market-based system of focused, coordinated care is having a profound effect on the values associated with health care. The emphasis of managed care organizations will be on wellness and health promotion, with pressure to decrease hospital care and costs (Hinitz-Satterfield et al., 1993). The new focus is on cost-efficient care that emphasizes management of chronic care issues rather than a primary focus on the management of acute-care problems. This changes the priorities of how resources are used. The emphasis is also on including a strong focus on outcomes, to determine effective care practices as well as the processes used in the delivery of care.

Changes Needed in the Health Care System

While the reforms in the health care delivery system are occurring, some other changes must also occur. There are a number of issues that are important to providing protection to the health care consumer. Hasan (1996) suggests that old ideas such as limitations placed by the health care provider concerning "preexisting health conditions" must be removed. There is also a need to develop methods to determine the effectiveness of treatments and find ways to guarantee coverage for all effective procedures. These are major problems and require open communication between health care researchers and managed care organizations. Another major issue is a means to prevent clinical decisions made on the basis of cost rather than medical need. This is related to finding ways to guard against providing incentives that result in underserving the enrolled population in the managed care organization.

In response to this problem, representatives from managed care organizations and physicians representing the American Medical Association have begun talks to look at the issue of "gag rules." These are rules placed upon the physicians by the managed care corporation in which restraints are placed on what treatment options can be discussed with patients. This is done to prevent the physician from discussing treatment procedures that are more costly than those the managed care organization prefers to provide. Federal legislation, as of January 1997, prevents a managed care organization from placing restrictions on discussion of treatment options by physicians. This is a start in the effort to find ways to protect third-party health consumers.

Another important need is for managed care organizations to find ways to manage chronic conditions to prevent escalation into the need for acute-care services. If managed care organizations are going to be cost effective, methods to manage enrolled members with chronic health conditions need to be developed. It is important to manage emerging problems before they require expensive in-hospital care. For example, managing enrolled members with diabetes mellitus so that their blood sugars remain within normal limits will ultimately save the health care organizations large amounts of money. Also, increased use of early diagnostic detection programs such as mammograms, cancer screening, and screening for high-risk pregnancy can be very cost effective. A goal of managed care organizations is to identify threats to health early so that expensive hospital treatment can be avoided.

Conclusions

Many of the goals of managed care health organizations are well in line with long-held goals of nursing. The use of health promotion and illness prevention strategies are highly valued by nurses. Thus, with these shared values, nurses can become important players in the managed care system. It is a time of great opportunity for nurses to demonstrate their effectiveness and to solidify their place in the health care system. They have the opportunity to demonstrate that nursing can contribute much to achieving the goals of managed care and thus provide for positive patient outcomes in a cost-effective manner.

References

Abbey, F. B. (1997). Health care reform: The road lies with managed care. In P. Kongstvedt (Ed.), *Essentials of managed health care* (2nd ed., pp. 17-35). Gaithersburg, MD: Aspen.

American Association of Retired Persons Special Bulletin. (1996, November). *Special report: Managed care.* Washington, DC: AARP.

Anderson, O. W. (1989). *The health services continuum in democratic states* (pp. 112-114). Ann Arbor, MI: Health Administration Press.

Bernstein, I. (1996). *Guns or butter: The presidency of Lyndon Johnson.* New York: Oxford University Press.

Coile, R. C. (1995). Advanced practice nurse: A critical resource for managed care. *Health Trends, 7*(7), 1-7.

Coppola, M. N., Croft, T., & Leo, E. (1997). Understanding the uninsured dilemma. *Medical Group Managment Journal, 44*(5), 72, 74, 76, 78-80, 82.

Curtin, L. (1994). Learning from the future. *Nursing Management, 25*(1), 7-9.

Ermann, D. (1988). Hospital utilization review: Past experience, future directions. *Journal of Health Politics, Policy, and Law, 13,* 683-704.

Friedman, E. A. (1996). End-stage renal disease therapy: An American success story. *Journal of the American Medical Association, 275*(14), 1118-1122.

Hasan, M. M. (1996). Let's end the nonprofit charade. *New England Journal of Medicine, 334*(16), 1055-1057.

Himali, U. (1995). Managed care: Does the promise meet the potential? *American Nurse, 27*(4), 14, 16.

Hinitz-Satterfield, P., Miller, E. H., & Hagan, E. P. (1993). Managed care and new roles for nursing: Utilization and case management in a health maintenance organization. In K. Kelly (Ed.), *Managing nursing care* (pp. 83-99). St. Louis, MO: Mosby.

Langston, T. S. (1992). *Ideologues and presidents: From the New Deal to the Reagan revolution.* Baltimore: Johns Hopkins University Press.

Long, M. J. (1994). *The medical care system: A conceptual model.* Ann Arbor, MI: Health Administration Press.

MacLeod, G. K. (1995). Overview of manged health care. In P. Kongstvedt (Ed.), *Essentials of managed health care* (pp. 1-9). Gaithersburg, MD: Aspen.

Menke, T. J. (1997). The effect of chain membership on hospital costs. *Health Services Research, 32*(2), 177-196.

Mezirow, J. (1994). Understanding transformation theory. *Adult Education Quarterly, 44*(4), 222-229.

Olsten Health. (1997). *21st century home care—Back to the future.* Retrieved September 3, 1998, from the World Wide Web: http://www.olstenhealth.com/indepth/homecare.htm

Rettig, R. A. (1996). The social contract and the treatment of permanent kidney failure. *Journal of the American Medical Association, 275*(14), 1123-1126.

Riley, D. W. (1994). Integrated health care systems: Emerging models. *Nursing Economics, 12*(4), 201-206.

Seattle Times. *Inflation drops, health care cost rises for workers.* Retrieved September 3, 1998, from the World Wide Web: http://archives.seattletimes.com/cgi-bin/texis/web/vortex/display?storyID16304

Sovie, M. D. (1995). Tailoring hospitals for managed care and integrated health systems. *Nursing Economics, 13*(2), 72-83.

Stevens, C. (1997). *Federally supported basic science research viewed as key to reducing cost and suffering from kidney disease.* Retrieved September 3, 1998, from the World Wide Web: http://www.asn-online.com/news/april2497.html

Turner, S. O. (1995, August). Reality check. *Hospitals and Health Networks, 69*(16), 20-22.

Venegoni, S. L. (1996). Changing environment of healthcare. In J. V. Hickey (Ed.), *Advanced practice nursing: Changing roles and clinical application* (pp. 77-90). Philadelphia: Lippincott.

Wagner, E. R. (1997). Types of managed care organizations. In P. Kongstvedt (Ed.), *Essentials of managed health care* (2nd ed., pp. 36-48). Gaithersburg, MD: Aspen.

Weissman, J. (1996). Uncompensated hospital care: Will it be there if we need it? *Journal of the American Medical Association, 27*(10), 823-828.

Chapter

2 Managed Care Organizational Structures

Margaret M. Conger

We would not be at the trouble to learn a language, if we could have all that is written in it just as well in translation.
—Samuel Johnson

For many entering the health care world as new providers, as well as for many who have long practiced under the old health care paradigm of fee for service, the language of the managed care world sounds like a foreign tongue. However, to be effective in this new world, it is necessary to master the new language. There are no easy translations. This chapter will introduce many of the terms and acronyms used in the managed care world. It is hoped that this introduction will help many to begin to speak this new language—or if not, at least know where to find the needed translations. Again, as Samuel Johnson has said, "Knowledge is of two kinds: we know a subject ourselves, or we know where we can find the information."

Managed care is a term used to describe both organizational structures that provide for the health needs of an enrolled population and various techniques used by health care organizations to control the costs of providing health care. The techniques often used include wellness promotion, health education, early identification of disease, incentives to providers for reducing cost of care, and a variety of utilization management strategies (Fox, 1997). The organizations that make use of these techniques can vary from a true health maintenance organization (HMO) to a variety of private health care insurance companies to federal government programs. This diversity of health care options in the United States has led to considerable confusion in the minds both of the public and of many health care providers. This chapter will attempt to bring some order out of the confusion that exists in understanding the multitude of health care organizations operating in this country. Also, the critical issues that need to be addressed as the American health care system moves toward the managed care environment will be considered. An understanding of these systems is needed to respond effectively in this new world of health care.

Description of Managed Care

A broad definition of managed care describes it as "any arrangement among health care providers, payers, and patients that offers incentives or imposes penalties designed to influence the utilization of medical services" (American Nurses Association, 1997). A desired outcome of managed care organizations is to provide health care at a low cost with increased efficiency by using effective management. There are several strategies used to attain this goal. First, services need to be provided in the most appropriate and least costly environment. Second, enrolled members in the plan need to be able to have early access to care so that health conditions do not worsen, requiring more expensive care. Third, the managed care organization needs to provide a continuum of services to cover a wide range of needs for potential enrolled members, from that of high-intensity acute care to health promotion and disease prevention services. If the managed care organization cannot provide for a health need of an enrolled member, it will need to go outside of the organization to secure the service, usually at increased cost. Finally, to be effective in managing health care costs, the organization must also be able to continuously conduct analysis and evaluation of utilization of services (Hinitz-Satterfield, Miller, & Hagan, 1993). Vigilant review of use of services is one important way to maintain close fiscal control.

Development of Managed Care Organizations

The rapid increase in the number of managed care organizations and the number of people receiving health care through this system is very recent in origin, but the foundations for this health delivery system go back into the early part of the 20th century. Health care organizations that were the forerunners of today's organizations started in the western part of the United States. The organization credited with being the first managed care health plan was developed in Tacoma, Washington: the Western Clinic (Fox, 1997). In 1929, a rural farmer's health cooperative was established in Oklahoma and was credited with establishing the first hospital associated with the health plan (Fox, 1997). The Kaiser Foundation Health Plan was started in 1937 to serve the needs of the workers and families employed by the Kaiser Construction Company. In all of these organizations, the enrolled member or his employer paid a small monthly fee to receive medical care. The term health maintenance organization (HMO) was coined by Paul Elwood, a physician advisor to President Nixon (Starr, 1982), to describe the early health care organizations such as the Kaiser system and the Group Health Cooperative of Puget Sound health care services.

Capitation Principles

Capitation is the payment method used by a managed care organization to finance its operation. In this system, a person or his or her employer pays a set monthly fee that covers most health care services. Based on the plan contract, the enrolled member may also pay various supplemental costs (copayments). For example, the enrolled member will usually pay a small amount for an office visit and for each prescription. However, these copayments tend to be less than charged in the typical fee-for-service contract. Because the member of the HMO prepays for services without regard to the type or number of services rendered, there is a great deal of safety for the member. The HMO assumes full risk for each member's care. If the member's care exceeds the fee, the HMO must absorb the cost. If the cost of the member's care falls below the fee paid, the HMO keeps the difference. This type of arrangement provides an incentive for the HMO to focus on preventive care so that enrolled members remain healthy.

The capitated payment system is a radical departure from the more familiar fee for service that has been the primary health care payment structure during recent times. In the fee for service arrangement, payment is made by either the patient or the insurer for each visit or service provided. In such a system, an increase in services provides increased revenue. The health care providers, such as physicians, hospitals, and clinical laboratories, are able to increase profits by increasing services. This results in a system in which there is no reward for promoting preventive health care services because such an approach would reduce profits. Because health care services are largely paid for by third-party payers such as the government or insurance companies, the individual recipient of the health care services has no reason to seek a limit to the amount of service sought. However, the third-party payer is very interested in limiting the services provided. Each increase in health service is a loss to the payer (for instance, an insurance company). Their profits are decreased when use of services increases. Thus, the payers and the providers are driven by opposing motivations (Bodenheimer & Grumbach, 1995).

This conflict of purpose that exists between payers and providers in the fee-for-service environment sets up an adversarial relationship. The third-party payer, the insurance company, has sought ways to decrease use of services. Some of these strategies include the need for a second opinion prior to surgery, prior authorization for hospitalization, and increased copayments for services billed directly to the customer. However, in the fee-for-service environment, the provider profits by increased use of services. Therefore, there has been little incentive to reduce services. This all changes in the managed care system. Here, the HMO becomes both the provider and the payer, thus reducing the mixed motivation. Instead, there is increased motivation to promote wellness and reduce service use. Efficiency in care is also a major incentive in the HMO setting. An important strategy used by managed care organizations to promote efficient use of services is the use of a primary care provider who oversees all of the care of the enrolled member. This person is referred to as a gatekeeper, or the person who must authorize all aspects of care. This concept will be explored in greater depth in the next chapter.

Health Maintenance Organizational Structures

There are a great number of possible organizational structures included in the general term of managed care organizations. Perhaps the best known of these managed care structures is the health maintenance organization—the HMO.

This can exist in a variety of permutations, each with its own organizational structure and a variety of degrees of control over the health care providers who deliver the health care services. The differences are usually based on the arrangements between the HMO and the physicians and the other health care services, such as laboratories, outpatient facilities, and acute-care hospitals. The attributes of the various managed care organizations that can loosely be described as an HMO are depicted in Table 2.1.

Staff Model HMO

In the staff model, the physicians are employed directly by the HMO. They generally work under clinic-type arrangements and only see patients who are members of the HMO. This arrangement is often referred to as a "closed panel" model because only physicians employed by the HMO can participate in the routine care of members of the group. Depending on the size of the HMO, some referrals may need to be made to outside physicians for very specialized care. The HMO will then cover the cost of the referral. An example of a staff model HMO is the Group Health Cooperative of Puget Sound, based in Seattle, Washington.

In the staff model HMO, there is very close control over use of services because of the tight arrangement between the physicians and the HMO. Utilization review practices are effective because the physicians, as employees of the organization, are closely regulated. Incentives such as bonuses for meeting performance and productivity standards are often used to increase buy-in among the physicians for this tight control (Wagner, 1997).

One problem in attracting potential members for this type of arrangement is the limited choices for health care. Also, if the depth of service options is too limited, potential enrollees may not join. Another reason for not joining this type of HMO is a prior longstanding relationship with a physician who is not a member of the HMO. Often people do not want to change such physician relationships. Of course, this freedom of choice is only possible if the individual member is joining the HMO. When the HMO is selected by an employer as the sole provider for the organization, such individual preferences do not matter.

This type of HMO can also have problems if the array of speciality practices is too limited because of the need for extensive referrals outside the HMO. Each time a referral is made outside the HMO, that ability to control costs is decreased. Finally, this type of arrangement does not work well in

TABLE 2.1 Comparison of Attributes: Health Maintenance Organizations

Managed Care Organization	*Degree of Control Over Costs*	*Physician Relationship*	*Enrollee Relationship*
HMO—staff model	Tight control over practice	Employee of HMO	Can use only physicians employed by HMO
HMO—group model			
Closed	Tight control over practice	Contract exclusively with HMO	Can use only physicians employed by HMO
Independent	Less control over practice	Contract with HMO, but can see other patients	Can use only physicians employed by HMO
Network model	Uses capitation as a control mechanism	Contracts with several multi-speciality physician groups	Current physician may be a member of the group: allows for greater freedom of choice
IPA	Uses capitation as a control mechanism	Physicians can contract with HMO either independently or in groups	Current physician may be a member of the group: allows for greater freedom of choice

NOTE: HMO = health maintenance organization; IPA = Independent Practice Association.

rural areas because of the need to provide a full range of physician services in a central location. In a rural area with a smaller population base, it becomes too costly to provide adequate services. This is a major reason for the slow development of managed care organizations in rural areas.

Group Model

A less restrictive type of physician arrangement with an HMO is that of the group model. In this type of arrangement, the HMO contracts with groups of doctors who provide care on a capitation basis for enrolled plan members. The physicians remain employed by their group practice rather than the HMO. Depending on the contract, the physicians may be allowed to see patients other than just those who are members of the HMO. In the closed-model type of organizational structure, the physicians can only see members of the HMO. This type of arrangement between the HMO and physicians is very tight and thus the control by the HMO over physician practice is similar to that seen in the staff model previously discussed. An example of this type of arrangement is the Kaiser Foundation Health Plan, which contracts with the Permanente Medical Group for physician services. These physicians care for members of the HMO exclusively. The Kaiser Foundation Health Plan functions as the HMO and manages all aspects of member needs, such as marketing the plan, enrolling members, and providing utilization review services. It also administers the hospitals used by the HMO.

In the independent arrangement in which physician groups contract with an HMO to provide services to group members, but at the same time see private-pay patients, there is less control of physician practice by the HMO. In this model, the HMO contracts with an independent, multispeciality physician group to provide medical services for group members. An example of this type of model is the Geisinger Health Plan in Danville, Pennsylvania, in which the HMO contracts with the Geisinger Clinic to provide physician services.

An advantage to the HMO in using a group model for physician coverage is that the HMO does not have to provide capital outlay to set up the physician offices and provide salaries. These are the responsibility of the physician group. The disadvantages for the HMO are similar to those in the staff model arrangement. Because enrollees can only use the services of a contracted physician, some potential members may be deterred from joining the group. Physician choice is a long tradition in the United States that is hard to overcome.

Network Model

The network model is an even less restrictive HMO physician arrangement. In this type of arrangement, the HMO contracts with a number of physician group practices to provide medical services for group members. Multispeciality physician groups are particularly sought out because of the broad health care coverage they can provide. An example of this type of arrangement is the Health Insurance Plan of Greater New York.

An HMO that contracts with multispeciality groups of physicians has a strong marketing appeal. The possibility that a physician with whom the potential member is already associated is a member of the HMO provides an incentive to join the group. Cost control can still be maintained by the HMO by providing a set amount of money per member to the physician group. If referrals need to be made outside the contracted physician groups, the physician group must pick up the cost out of their capitated funds. Also, the HMO maintains control over health care facility use by requiring preauthorization for use of services.

Independent Practice Association

The least restrictive arrangement between physicians and HMOs is that of the independent practice association (IPA). In this arrangement, the physicians form an association that then contracts with the HMO. Each physician practices out of an independent office, either by him- or herself or with a small group. Each physician has the freedom to see both HMO patients and other fee-for-service patients. Some IPA groups limit the physician members to practicing in only one hospital; others have physician groups that use several hospitals in a community.

Again, the payment arrangement for physicians in the IPA is that of capitation. The HMO pays the IPA a set amount for each member of the HMO who has selected a particular physician practice as the primary provider. The IPA pays the physicians, either in a fee-for-service arrangement or on a capitated plan based on the number of members for which each physician is responsible.

This type of loose structure is often the first step in moving toward tighter control. In rural areas where the potential patient volume is not sufficient to warrant a full time HMO, this arrangement will often be developed. It allows the HMO to contract with independent physicians to see members of the HMO without a large outlay of capital. It is also very attractive to potential HMO members because of the breadth of possible physician choices. However, because of the looseness of the connection of the HMO and the individual physician, it is the most difficult type of relationship in terms of maintaining control over cost and use of services.

Alternate Types of Managed Care Arrangements

Although all health care organizations use some of the managed care principles, there are some types of organizational structures that are less restrictive for both physicians and enrollees than those discussed in the previous section. The attributes of these organizations are depicted in Table 2.2.

TABLE 2.2 Comparison of Attributes: Less-Structured Managed Care Organizations

Managed Care Organization	*Degree of Control Over Costs*	*Physician Relationship*	*Enrollee Relationship*
PPO	Control over cost is less than in traditional HMO	Contracts to provide services at discounted rates	Wide selection of physicians–requires higher co-pay if uses non-contracted physician
EPO	Increased control over costs	Contracts to provide services at discounted rates	Required to use contracted physician
PHO	Enter into capitation arrangements with HMO	Physician and hospital form alliance to control practice	Wide selection of physicians–requires higher co-pay if uses non-contracted physician
Physician network	Group retains control over costs	Physicians control own practice	Must use contracted physicians

NOTE: EPO = exclusive provider organization; HMO = health maintenance organization; PPO = preferred provider organization; PHO = physician-hospital organization.

Preferred Provider Organization

The preferred provider organization (PPO) is a fee-for-service type of organizational structure in which members are provided with health care services from contracted providers. These arrangements are generally made between the insuring group—often an employer-sponsored health plan—and the participating physician groups. A preferred provider organization consists of a network of independent physicians and hospitals that contract to provide services at discounted rates. An arrangement such as this provides more choices to the group members than does the typical HMO organization but results in less coordination of care and thus reduced control over costs.

Contracted physicians, laboratory services, physical and occupational services, and other health services develop an agreement with the PPO to provide their services at a discounted rate. These providers agree to charging at a preestablished fee schedule. In return for providing the services at a discounted rate, the provider is guaranteed an increased patient load. The PPO benefits by securing health care services at less than the going rate for the community, and the physician is guaranteed a steady volume of patients.

The enrolled members in the PPO are given a discounted price for services received as long as they use the providers approved by the agency. If a group participant goes outside of the approved provider list, a higher copayment schedule is required. Because of the loose arrangement between the PPO and the physician group, very intensive utilization management practices are needed to control costs. A great emphasis is placed on preauthorization of services. Also, intense management of acute-care hospital stays and outpatient services is typically found in this type of organization.

Exclusive Provider Organization

Another type of fee for service managed care structure is the exclusive provider organization (EPO). This is very similar to the PPO structure except that it is more stringent in managing member choices. The group participants are required to use the physician groups that have been contracted with. If a group participant uses services provided by a nonmember provider, that care will not be paid for. This type of arrangement is generally developed between a large employer and a physician and hospital network. Because the members are captive, that is, are dependent upon their employer for health care coverage, the employer can be successful in arranging such a controlled arrangement.

Physician-Hospital Organization

The physician-hospital organization (PHO) is a form of organizational structure in which hospitals and physicians come together to market their resources. In this arrangement, physicians and hospitals form an alliance to negotiate contracts with either a managed care organization or large employer group. A capitation type of payment system is used. Physician membership in the organization can be either open or closed. In an open situation, virtually all physician members of the hospital's medical staff may join. In a closed arrangement, physician membership is limited by either speciality practice or a proven record of cost and quality effectiveness. Because of the large number of physicians involved in the practice, enrolled members have a wide selection of physicians and can often maintain a long-standing relationship with a physician of choice.

The advantage of a PHO is the increased strength of position when negotiating with the managed care organization to achieve a more lucrative contract than could be done on an independent basis. This could, of course, backfire if the managed care organization has the means to get contracts with other groups at better rates. A number of large employee unions are also looking at this type of arrangement in an effort to control the administrative costs present in some for-profit HMOs. A PHO arrangement is also common in situations in which a managed care organization is just coming into a market area and finds it more expedient to contract with a single group rather than a multitude of physician and hospital groups.

This type of arrangement, however, is being shown to have limited success in markets where there is strong managed care competition (Wagner, 1997). Wagner suggests that a managed care organization may not want to give up some of its control over cost management to another organization if it has sufficient client population to warrant managing its own system. Thus, this organizational structure will continue to be used primarily in rural areas where the potential population for membership in a managed care organization is limited (Wagner, 1997).

Physician Network

Another possible arrangement for health care coverage is for a group of doctors who work together to accept financial risk for covering enrolled persons without going through a third-party intermediary such as an insurance company. This is called a physician network. This arrangement avoids the cost of paying the insurance company for services; of course, the network will pick up the management costs directly. This organizational structure provides for greater autonomy for physicians than in other types of managed care. However, the choices for enrolled members are limited to those physicians under contract by the organization.

The movement of physicians into groups such as this is escalating as backlash against some of the tight fiscal controls of HMOs has increased. Examples of such groups include the University of California, Los Angeles Medical Group in the Los Angeles area; and the Doctors Care Plan in Washington, DC. A prime reason for this movement is that physicians are attempting to regain control over medical decision making rather than having decisions controlled by business people not versed in medicine. These groups may then contract with an HMO to cover their patients, but the control for the health care decisions remains with the physicians.

Elements of Financial Risk

In each of the health provider organizational plans, the concept of who is at financial risk must always be considered. In the traditional fee-for-service plan, the primary risk taker was the insurance company responsible for "paying the bill." The physician or hospital, as the provider of care, had no risk. All services were billed for, and thus there was no reason to limit services (Kongstvedt, 1997). This has, of course, changed radically in recent years; the payer organizations have become more proactive. The advent of the DRG system began to change who took financial risk. With an amount of money allocated prospectively to cover the cost of providing care in a hospital, part of the financial risk was redistributed. The hospital assumed major financial loss if the needed care was not provided efficiently (Health Care Financing Administration, 1994). However, in the DRG system, the physician provider did not face financial risk, and this resulted in a conflict of interest between the hospital and physician about how much care should be provided. The element of financial risk in the traditional fee-for-service plan—a retrospective plan—as compared to the risk for a prospective plan is shown in Figure 2.1. As can be seen, under the prospective plan, the provider (the hospital) and the payer are more equal. But note that in both systems the risk for the physician is very small.

At the extreme other end of the continuum of organizational plans, the staff model HMO takes all of the financial risk (Kongstvedt, 1997). Each member is charged a given fee per month, paid either by the employer or, if the member is not on an employee plan, by that member. In return, the member is guaranteed provision of all appropriate health care. The relationships of financial risk in various HMO models are shown in Figure 2.2. In the staff-model HMO, the physicians are salaried employees of the HMO and thus take virtually no risk. However, their income may be affected by a decrease of profit if their productivity falls below an expected level (Wagner, 1997).

In the group, network, and IPA models of HMOs, the risk is shared between the HMO and the group of physicians who have contracted to provide

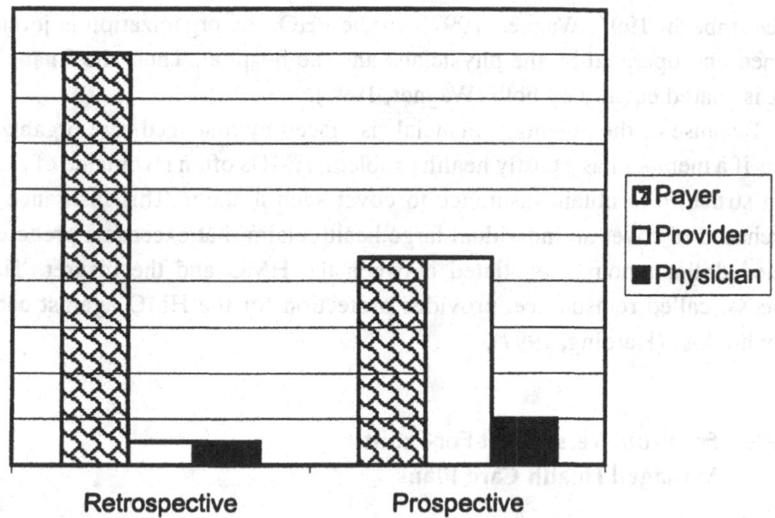

Figure 2.1 Comparison of Financial Risk: Fee for Service

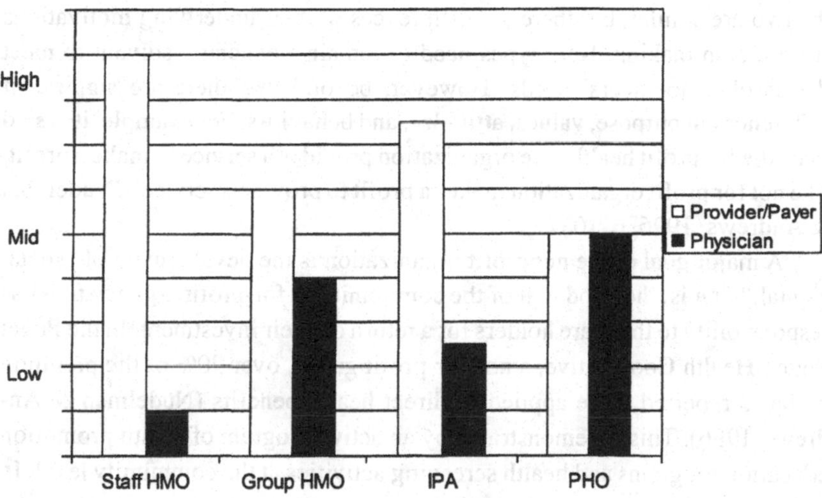

Figure 2.2 Comparison of Financial Risk: HMO Plans

care. The HMO will accept risk in all aspects of care other than physician services. The physicians take on the risk of being able to provide an acceptable level of medical services for the amount of money contracted (Bodenheimer

& Grumbach, 1995; Wagner, 1997). In the PHO, the organization is jointly owned and operated by the physicians and the hospital. Thus, the financial risk is shared equally by both (Wagner, 1997).

Because of the potential financial risk faced by managed care organizations if a member has a costly health problem, HMOs often go outside of their own structure to obtain insurance to cover such a claim. This insurance is purchased to cover an individual large health claim that exceeds a predetermined dollar amount negotiated between the HMO and the insurer. This process, called reinsurance, provides protection for the HMO against catastrophic loss (Harding, 1997).

For-Profit Versus Not-For-Profit Managed Health Care Plans

Another issue that needs to be addressed is the difference between managed health care plans that are for profit and those that are not. The structures of the two are similar, but there are differences in their underlying motivations for decision making. Both types need to remain financially solvent to meet the enrolled members' needs. However, beyond that there are significant differences in purpose, values, attitudes, and behaviors. For example, it is said that "the for profit health care organization provides a service to make a profit. The not for profit organization makes a profit to provide a service" (Nudelman & Andrews, 1996, p. 1057).

A major goal of the nonprofit organization is the development of "social capital," that is, the good will of the community. A for-profit organization has responsibility to the share holders for a return on their investment. In the Puget Sound Health Cooperative, a not-for-profit group, over 90% of the premium dollar is reported to be applied to direct health benefits (Nudelman & Andrews, 1996). This is demonstrated by an active program of health promotion education programs and health screening activities at the community level. In contrast to this, the usual profit returned to the consumer in health care services in the for-profit sector of managed care is about 70% to 80%.

Some providers associated with the for-profit sector suggest that comparisons such as these are not valid (Hasan, 1996). They claim that one cannot compare the percentage of premium dollars returned to the consumer in terms of health care services between the two types of organizations. Within the for-profit sector, a significant portion of the earned money is paid back to the community in taxes; in the not-for-profit organization, there is no return of tax to the community. Also, the for-profit organizations have different marketing and educational needs and thus cannot be compared financially to the nonprofit organization. Hasan suggests that this is an argument that may not be resolved easily. It may well be that the consumer will determine which type is most effective in meeting health care needs by selecting the HMO that provides the highest quality of service at the lowest cost.

Hasan (1996) also suggests that it is appropriate for the for-profit and not-for-profit organizations to have differences in mission. The mission of the not-for-profit organization is to meet the social needs of the community, such as caring for the indigent, providing an educational role for health profession students at all levels, and carrying out medical research. This should be done in return for the tax advantages provided to the not-for-profit organizations. The for-profit organization needs to focus on payback to the stockholders to keep the organization viable. Its social responsibility is managed through the payment of tax on the corporation's profit.

Federally Financed HMOs

The federal government has also encouraged the expansion of HMO development by providing financial funding for two special groups of potential HMO enrollees. Both Medicare and Medicaid recipients are being encouraged to enroll in specially developed managed care organizations. The shift of Medicare recipients into an HMO-type structure from the traditional fee-for-service plans has accelerated rapidly. It is estimated that there were 80,000 new enrollees in an HMO per month during 1996 ("Senior surge," 1997). The funds that provide the enrollment fees for these Medicare recipients come from the Health Care Financing Administration (HCFA).

Medicare HMO

The availability of HMO plans for the Medicare population has accelerated, under considerable encouragement from the federal government. In this arrangement, the HMO plan contracts with HCFA to receive money that normally would be used to pay for fee-for-service contracts. The HMO contracts with HCFA on a yearly basis and, during that time, cannot change rates charged to the enrolled members or reduce any of the contracted services. The amount of money the HMO receives for each enrollee is presently calculated at 95% of what has been determined to be the actual cost of medical services if they had been obtained through a usual fee-for-service plan (Zarabozo & LeMasurier, 1995). However, this percentage is under considerable debate and could well be lowered in the near future. Any lowering of the amount of money provided to the HMO will probably alter the amount of services that will be provided.

Because of regional differences in health care costs, the amount of money received varies from one location to another. An HMO located in an area with a pattern of high Medicare cost per enrollee is allocated more money than a region in which the cost per enrollee is lower. In addition to the money paid by HCFA, each enrolled member in the Medicare HMO also pays the Part B coverage directly to the HMO. As part of the agreement with HFCA, the Medicare HMO must provide all of the normal Medicare-covered services. Some Medicare HMOs charge an additional monthly fee over and above the Medicare Part B payment to provide additional services not required by government standards. Common additional services include such items as partial payment of prescriptions and eyeglasses not covered by the fee-for-service Medicare plan. The additional services are an important marketing tool for the HMO and have encouraged Medicare members to frequently move from one HMO to another.

To be eligible to receive a contract with HCFA, an HMO must demonstrate that it has the ability to offer all Medicare services such as hospitals, skilled nursing facilities, and home health services. It must also be able to provide emergency services. HCFA screens potential Medicare HMOs carefully because the enrollment pattern of the Medicare HMO is quite different from that of employer-sponsored enrolled groups. In the Medicare HMO, each member is enrolled individually, rather than as a group, as happens with employer-sponsored plans. This type of enrollment leads to two possible problems. First, the marketing strategies for the Medicare HMO are more costly than for employer-sponsored groups because of the need to sign up each member individually. There is concern that money spent on marketing may reduce health care services. The other problem is that because there is no employer looking out for the welfare of the participants such as there is in employer-sponsored groups, the number and quality of services may be reduced. To ensure the quality of the services offered by the HMO, HCFA must take on a monitoring role.

The success of the Medicare HMO movement has been mixed. A report by Cher and Lenert (1997) suggests that in a 4-year study, older people and poor people were more than twice as likely to decline in health in an HMO as in a traditional plan, a fee-for-service arrangement. There is a mixed reaction to this report. The question is whether the enrollees avoid prolonged costly care and thus die more mercifully, as claimed by Cher and Lenert, or if the quality of care is reduced by not giving the patients and their families options that could prolong life (Curtis & Rubenfeld, 1997). Another problem among the Medicare HMOs is that the enrollees have used more services than had been originally projected (Zarabazo & LeMasurier, 1997). This has made many of the Medicare HMOs unprofitable and has resulted in a decline in the number of such plans available. Thus, there are many questions that need to be answered about the effectiveness of the Medicare HMO in meeting the health needs of the elderly population.

Another issue for many Medicare beneficiaries, when deciding to stay in a traditional fee-for-service plan or switch to an HMO, is the issue of travel. A common phenomenon of the American culture is the migration of retirees from the cold north to the sunbelt areas of the United States every winter. If a person is locked into an HMO service area that inhibits such travel, there is a disinclination to join the HMO. Thus, there is a great need for Medicare HMOs to develop more flexible plans to attract the potential members who live part of the year away from their home base. A point-of-service-type contract is an emerging form of HMO service plan that addresses this issue. In this type of plan, the enrolled member can receive health care up to a certain percentage of the total health care costs outside of the HMO-approved providers. Provision of care in an out-of-state site has a number of difficulties related to the ability of the parent organization to provide insurance coverage in another state. The growth of multistate HMO structures will help in solving this problem (Carneal, 1997).

Medicaid HMO

The Medicaid program was established to cover the health care costs of the poor. Its success in meeting this goal has been marginal. Technically, all persons who fall under the federal poverty level guidelines are eligible for assistance with health care—the reality is that few states have actually provided services for this entire population. Nationally, the average income for persons who qualify for the Medicaid program is less than half of the federal poverty level standard (Rooks, 1990). In an attempt to provide better coverage to the poor, a movement to increase the number of Medicaid programs that use a managed care system is emerging.

More than 36 million low-income persons in the United States receive health care through a Medicaid managed care plan (Rooks, 1990). This movement began in California in the early 1970s when the state began to contract with HMOs to provide indigent care (American Nurses Association, 1997). Arizona also developed an alternative plan to the usual fee-for-service arrangement for providing health care to the indigent when it began its program for indigent health care. This plan, the Arizona Health Care Cost Containment System (AHCCCS), used a managed care approach for its delivery system.

To develop an HMO-type program, a state must secure a waiver from the federal government to provide a plan in which the enrollee's freedom to choose a provider is limited to a managed care structure only. Federal legislation requires that Medicaid recipients have the chance to choose between a fee-for-service health plan and a managed care health plan. Before a state can develop a plan to move Medicaid recipients from a fee-for-service plan into a managed care plan, it must apply for a Freedom of Choice Waiver 1915(b).

Other states are also moving rapidly in the direction of developing managed care Medicaid programs. Tennessee has recently moved into a managed care arrangement called TennCare (Meyer, 1996). The Tennessee program allows for all state residents who are at 100% or lower of the federal poverty guideline to enroll in the program. This program also provides the opportunity for all state residents earning up to 400% of the federal poverty guideline to enroll on a sliding scale fee basis. This provision is making health care benefits available to many of the working poor (Meyer, 1996).

Other states with a large managed care program for the Medicaid population are Hawaii and Oregon. The Oregon program has engendered considerable debate with its attempt to develop a list of services ranked in priority that would be provided under the Medicaid program. The legislature would then determine the amount of money that would be funded for the program. Using this information, a determination of the services that would be provided would be directly tied to the amount of money allocated for health care (Bodenheimer & Grumbach, 1995).

For a state to develop a Medicaid managed health care plan, it must meet some very specific guidelines. First, the plan must include a means to perform a health status and a risk assessment for enrolled members. Second, it must demonstrate progress in developing health promotion and disease prevention programs. Third, it must provide care using an interdisciplinary team approach. Fourth, the plan must provide a primary care gatekeeper for all enrolled members and have a strong utilization management plan in place.

There are a number of considerations that should be included when a state elects to develop a managed care structure for its Medicaid population (Meyer, 1996). Most important, there must be effective communication with community leaders who can demonstrate understanding and acceptance of the plan. Without this communication, there is great danger of total chaos. The situation that occurred during the initial years of the TennCare program serves as a good example. In Tennessee, development of the TennCare program happened so quickly that neither community leaders nor health care providers were kept apprised of the changes. This resulted in several years of confusion, with an uneven balance between the providers available and the consumers' needs (Meyer, 1996). It is important for the managed care organization to demonstrate that there is sufficient access to health care resources in all parts of the state where the plan will be used.

The organization must also demonstrate the ability to provide effective utilization management practices, and it must have financial stability so the health care needs of the enrollees will be met. As with all government-sponsored programs, strong regulatory practices will be used to ensure that enrolled members are receiving adequate health care. In the TennCare program, these guidelines were not followed, acocunting for some of the problems the program experienced when it tried to rapidly move 100% of its eligible Medicaid population into the managed care environment (Meyer, 1996). The infrastructure to provide services was not in place to meet the needs of the members in the early years.

Other Federally Financed Health Programs

Veterans Affairs Program

In addition to the Medicare and Medicaid programs financed directly by federal money, the Veterans Affairs (formerly Veterans Administration) program is another example of government-sponsored health care. It provides health care to eligible veterans through 173 hospitals, 133 nursing homes, and

40 domiciliaries (Gillies, Shortell, & Young, 1997). This health care system is facing the same economic constraints as all other health care providers and is attempting to restructure itself into a more cost-efficient organization while maintaining quality care. It has recently restructured itself into 22 networks of care in an effort to better coordinate the health needs of the veterans it serves.

A major problem facing the Veterans Administration Health Services is the aging and thus increased health needs of its population. It is also facing a decrease in revenues due to its decreasing population (Gillies et al., 1997). To meet these challenges, it is trying to increase its use of managed care principles, such as better coordination of services, increasing its focus on health promotion, and improving quality in an effort to retain its users. Its movement from a system that focused on acute hospital care to one that focuses on health promotion in community settings will be a major challenge.

Indian Health Service

Another federally funded health care program is the Indian Health Service, an agency of the Public Health Service. Provision of health service to Native Americans (including Alaska Natives) has arisen out of written treaties going back to the 19th century (Kunitz, 1996). Money is appropriated by the federal government to provide health care based on census data reflecting the number of people living on reservation lands. All people who hold proof of tribal affiliation are eligible for care (Goldsmith, 1996).

The Indian Health system also receives support from other federal programs in that is a "residual provider" (Goldsmith, 1996, p. 1788). This means that if a tribal member has other health care insurance, those resources must be used before money allocated to the IHS is used. Because of the high level of poverty found on many reservations, many tribal members using the IHS qualify for Medicaid programs. Thus the IHS is really funded by both Medicaid monies and federal appropriations (Goldsmith, 1996). Despite these funding sources, the total monetary outlay per person for health care is about 60% to 65% of that spent per person on a national level (Kunitz, 1996).

The IHS has long been a highly integrated health service, with clinics, field stations, and public health services all linked to a general hospital. In fact, it has been a model of a well-run affordable program; some have suggested that it could have been used as a model for the Clinton health reform program (Jorgensen, 1996). However, the movement in the 1990s has been to break up this highly integrated system and return control of health care to tribal authorities. It is feared by some that this will increase costs because each tribal group will have to go outside its own health care system to purchase care that it does not have sufficient call for. This could, in the long run, lead to expensive, fragmented programs (Kunitz, 1996).

The Indian Health Service, then, has been developed as an early model of a managed care organization. Whether it will retain this organizational structure remains to be seen. If the current trends continue, there is concern that it will become merged with other managed care organizations and lose its unique place as a service to Alaska Natives and other Native Americans (Goldsmith, 1996; Jorgensen, 1996).

Conclusions

Managed care organizations are becoming the predominant health care delivery system in the United States. Their emphasis on delivering cost-effective care and retaining quality goals has a direct impact on the delivery of nursing care. Nurses need to learn the language of the managed care environment to be successful in finding their place in this movement.

This chapter has introduced a description of managed care organizations and differentiated between the various types. The issue of who is at financial risk in the various types of arrangements aids in understanding the basis of health care decisions. This understanding of financial risk is important when advocating for patients who need health care. It is far more productive to work with the managed care system to aid in achieving the dual objectives of cost effectiveness and quality care rather than just complain about the changes that have occurred.

The movement of government-sponsored programs into the managed care environment is projected to increase because it is seen as an important solution to the management of monetary deficits in health care programs for the elderly. The nurse needs to understand how both the Medicare and Medicaid programs function to serve as an educator for the many people who are having to make a choice between a managed care provider and a fee-for-service plan. The future of both the government-sponsored Veterans Administration Health System and the Indian Health Service are in question. These programs also need to shift into a managed care mode for their survival.

Nurses need to be involved in these restructuring processes. To do this, they need to learn the language. The information in this chapter is designed to help the nurse do just that.

References

American Nurses Association. (1997). *Report to the House of Delegates.* Retrieved September 3, 1998, from the World Wide Web: http://www.ana.org/gova/hod97/mgcare.htm

Bodenheimer, T. S., & Grumbach, K. (1995). *Understanding health policy: A clinical approach.* Norwalk, CT: Appleton & Lange.

Carneal, G. (1997). State regulation of managed care. In P. Kongstvedt (Ed.), *Essentials of managed health care* (2nd ed., pp. 453-469). Gaithersburg, MD: Aspen.

Cher, D., & Lenert, L. (1997). Method of Medicare reimbursement and the rate of potentially ineffective care of critically ill patients. *Journal of the American Medical Association, 278*(12), 1000-1007.

Curtis, R., & Rubenfeld, G. (1997). Aggressive medical care at the end of life. *Journal of the American Medical Association, 278*(12), 1025-1026.

Fox, P. D. (1997). An overview of managed care. In P. Kongstvedt (Ed.), *Essentials of managed health care* (2nd ed., pp. 3-16). Gaithersburg, MD: Aspen.

Gillies, R., Shortell, S., & Young, G. (1997). Best practices in managing organized delivery systems. *Hospital & Health Services Administration, 42*(3), 299-321.

Goldsmith, M. F. (1996). First Americans face their latest challenge: Indian health care meets state Medicaid reform. *Journal of the American Medical Association, 275*(23), 1786-1788.

Harding, D. F. (1997). Operational finance and budgeting. In P. Kongstvedt (Ed.), *Essentials of managed health care* (2nd ed., pp. 352-365). Gaithersburg, MD: Aspen.

Hasan, M. M. (1996). Let's end the nonprofit charade. *New England Journal of Medicine, 334*(16), 1055-1057.

Health Care Financing Administration. (1994). *Refinement of the Medicare diagnosis related groups to incorporate a measure of severity.* Retrieved September 3, 1998, from the World Wide Web: http://www.irpsys.com/srdrg.htm

Hinitz-Satterfield, P., Miller, E. H., & Hagan, E. P. (1993). Managed care and new roles for nursing: Utilization and case management in a health maintenance organization. In K. Kelly (Ed.), *Managing nursing care* (pp. 83-99). St. Louis, MO: Mosby.

Jorgensen, J. G. (1996). Comment: Recent twists and turns in American Indian health care. *American Journal of Public Health, 86*(10), 1362-1364.

Kongstvedt, P. R. (1997). Compensation of primary care physicians in open panel plans. In P. Kongstvedt (Ed.), *Essentials of managed health care* (2nd ed., pp. 115-137). Gaithersburg, MD: Aspen.

Kunitz, S. J. (1996). The history and politics of US health care policy for American Indians and Alaskan Natives. *American Journal of Public Health, 86*(10), 1464-1473.

Meyer, G. S. (1996). TennCare and academic medical centers. *Journal of the American Medical Association, 276*(9), 672-676.

Nudelman, P. M., & Andrews, L. M. (1996). The "value added" of not-for-profit health plans. *New England Journal of Medicine, 334*(16), 1057-1059.

Rooks, J. P. (1990). Let's admit we ration health care—then set priorities. *American Journal of Nursing, 90*(6), 39-43.

Senior surge: Are you ready? (1997). *Hospital and Health Networks, 71*(7), 50-56.

Starr, P. (1982). *The social transformation of American medicine*. New York: Basic Books.

Wagner, E. R. (1997). Types of managed care organizations. In P. R. Kongstvedt (Ed.), *Essentials of managed health care* (2nd ed., pp. 36-48). Gaithersburg, MD: Aspen.

Zarabozo, C., & LeMasurier, J. D. (1995). Medicare and managed care. In P. R. Kongstvedt (Ed.), *Essentials of managed health care* (2nd ed., pp. 405-431). Gaithersburg, MD: Aspen.

Chapter

3 Managed Care Organizational Strategies Used to Achieve Organizational Goals

Margaret M. Conger

> ***For it's all in some language I don't know. . . . Why, it's a looking-glass book, of course! And if I hold it up to the glass, the words will all go the right way again.***
>
> Alice (in Lewis Carroll's ***Through the Looking Glass***)

Health care in the United States is in the midst of evolution. The paradigm shift occurring is one described as a second-order change, in which the underlying value systems are totally altered. In a second-order change of this magnitude, the value system will never revert to the former system. To be successful in this new environment, one must have a way to understand these new values. As Alice found when she stepped into the looking-glass room, she needed to hold the book up to a looking-glass to turn the words around so she could read them. Nurses, too, need to turn their focus around to read the new worldview.

This chapter will attempt to serve as a mirror to help nurses understand the values inherent in this new health care system. The goals of managed care organizations will be explained. This will then set the foundation for the second section of the book, in which nursing's response to the shift of values that are occurring in health care will be examined.

To meet the dual goals of managed care—cost-effectiveness and quality care—management strategies must be altered. These strategies include the need for integration of services, coordination of care, new health promotion strategies, and means to carry out quality management. In this chapter, these strategies will be explored and their importance to the managed care environment will be analyzed.

Integration of Services

Integration of health care services is an important strategy used in successful managed care organizations. Shortell, Gillies, Anderson, Erickson, and Mitchell (1996) describe integration of health care services as a process in which all of an organization's activities are coordinated or blended to provide a functional structure. This blending of a myriad of services is necessary if the goal of cost effectiveness is to be achieved. At least theoretically, a decided benefit of integration of multiple health services into one larger organization is the effect of economy of scale. A large organization has a competitive edge over a smaller one in terms of buying power, negotiating contracts, and other such activities. Also, with a large base of health services to work from, clinical resources can be deployed in a more cost-effective manner, leading to less duplication of services (Menke, 1997). As the clinical services of health care organizations in a geographic area are combined into one organization, there can be a reduction in duplication of services such as diagnostic testing, clinical laboratories, and health promotion activities.

Also, when services are combined in a larger organization, a greater ability to influence health provider behavior is expected. A large organization can exert control over the providers more effectively than when each provider is working independently. Such influence is vital to achieving the cost effectiveness goals of managed care. Kongstvedt and Plocher (1995) state that the greatest cost control measure in health care is the ability to influence medical utilization. Only by reducing unnecessary medical procedures will true health care costs be reduced.

At the larger level, health services in a community need to be integrated within the organization so that acute tertiary care, subacute care, long-term care, and primary care can all be provided. In an integrated system such as this, a patient is able to stay within the same organization, thus reducing the need for referrals to agencies outside of the system. In this way, the organization retains control over the entire continuum of care and can thus reduce cost. This concept of integrated services is a far cry from the fee-for-service era, when every hospital saw neighboring institutions as competitors for the potential customer and each strove to entice the potential customer with its services. In the managed care environment, duplication of services in close proximity is not cost-effective.

However, even in an integrated system, some duplication of services is needed. In a study by Shortell et al. (1996), it was found necessary to have more than one site delivering the same service within the system to deal with demands over the geographic area. The health care organization must be very conscious of the distance a client is willing to travel to obtain service. For example, in a large metropolitan area, people were unwilling to travel into the center of the city to receive minor services. It was necessary, therefore, for the health care organization to provide preventive and maintenance services in convenient locations scattered throughout the metropolitan area.

The health care industry is also highly dependent on the integration of services because of the nature of its work. There is a need for a high degree of reciprocal interdependence between providers (Shortell et al., 1996). Reciprocal interdependence is a situation in which two groups need to exchange resources in an ongoing fashion for each to be successful. For example, physicians are highly dependent on other resources, such as pharmacies to provide needed medications, clinical laboratories to provide needed data, nurses to manage care, and a myriad of other such services. None of these providers can do their job without interaction with the others. For each of these providers to be successful, a high degree of integration is needed.

In the health care industry, three types of integration exist (Shortell et al., 1996). The first, *functional integration*, means bringing together the key support services of a health care organization such as financial management, human resource management, and long-range planning services. The second type is *clinical integration*, in which patient services are well coordinated. The third is *physician system integration*, in which a physician's practice is closely allied with the services of the parent organization (Gillies, Shortell, & Young, 1997). Each of these types of integration will be addressed.

Functional Integration

Functional integration involves the coordination of important support services used by all of the agencies of the parent organization. Management systems used to control finances, such as the budgeting and accounting systems, need to be integrated. Also needed is the long-range planning function, which includes input from all of the stakeholders of the organization. Representatives from the primary care sites located throughout the community, the subacute facilities, and the tertiary care hospital need to be included in this planning function. Also needed is a well-integrated communication system. The use of advanced technology such as computers for sharing and storing client information and fax machines to speed the transfer of information from one site to another is necessary. There must be a smooth transfer of information and records between each of the subunits of the organization. The patient record from an in-hospital stay must be available at all other levels of care, such as the home health agency or the primary care site, to expedite care.

Shared databases for information pertaining to the structure of the organization are also useful. For example, shared human resources data can be helpful in placing the most appropriate employee in the correct job. Finally, the quality management system must cut across all levels of care. Integration of these functions will result in the greatest value for the system (Gillies et al., 1997).

Clinical Integration

Clinical integration refers to the arrangement in which the multitude of health care services is brought together under a combined structure. Such an arrangement reduces costly duplication of services and provides the opportunity for professionals to learn from each other. For example, the use of computer-based information has been shown to eliminate duplicate testing and procedures (Shortell et al., 1996).

In the study by Shortell et al. (1996) in which 11 health care systems were examined, those whose facilities were geographically in proximity were more successful in integrating services. Well-coordinated networks were most successful in urban areas where facilities were close to each other. However, in rural areas, such integration of services was found to be a problem. The study showed that systems that had greater than a 50-mile distance between facilities rated lower on the clinical integration scale (Shortell et al., 1996). It was difficult to share clinical service lines, support services, and personnel because of the limits as to how far clients were willing to travel to get needed health services. Communication between providers was also more restricted.

Physician System Integration

Physician integration into the health care system may be the most difficult to achieve because of the long history of independent physician practice. The goal of cost-effective care is hard to achieve when physicians are working in independent practices (Kongstvedt, 1995; Shortell et al., 1996). The historical working arrangement of physicians has been in solo practice or small groups. However, to achieve the goals of managed care organizations, it is necessary for physicians to work in larger groups than were common in the "cottage industry" period. Physicians appear to be more likely to move into group working relationships in situations that are familiar to them. In other words, a group that arises out of a hospital working relationship is more likely to be successful than a group that is formed from physicians with no prior relationship to each other.

Integration is also needed when planning for quality management of clinical conditions. Common protocols need to be developed for a fully integrated system to be successful. This is particularly important in managing patients with chronic illness. At the local unit, physicians need to agree on specific treatment protocols so that persons receiving care at two different sites receive comparable care. To achieve this type of integration, the providers within the managed care organization in a geographical area need to come together to share knowledge, costs, risks and rewards and develop standardized protocols (Shortell et al., 1996).

Coordination of Care

One of the positive outcomes of an integrated health care system that can be achieved with managed care is that of increased continuity of care. For example, in the fee-for-service system, a patient may be seen by a number of health care providers who are not in communication with each other. It is not unusual for a patient to receive prescriptions from several physicians, each with no knowledge of what the other has ordered. It is hoped that with the movement into managed care, the coordination problem can be better managed. In the study by Shortell et al. (1996), such redundancy in care was reduced when one physician was better aware of the goals of other care providers.

Limitations on Selection of Providers

There are several strategies common to all health maintenance organizations used to coordinate care. One important strategy is to limit the choice of enrolled members in the selection of a physician provider. The physicians and health services provided by the HMO organization are generally the only ones available to the member. If the member chooses to go outside of the HMO for services, the charges for the service become the financial responsibility of the member. The flexibility to choose care outside of the HMO varies among health plans. Some will not allow members to seek treatment outside of the health plan. An important strategy of an HMO is to develop a large pool of patients so the costs of more expensive patients can be spread over the entire pool. Allowing members to seek services outside the contracted network dilutes the control the HMO has in controlling costs.

The use of the limited choice of providers has come under considerable debate (Miller, 1997). There are increased questions about whether or not this practice actually promotes continuity of care because of both the frequent movement of enrollees from one plan to another and the frequency in which physicians move from one plan to another. Recent legislation at the state level has begun to address this issue. A number of states have passed legislation that allows the enrollee to request continuance of care for a limited time with a provider who is not a member of the managed care organization (Miller, 1997). The reason a change in physician provider is required could arise from either a change in managed care organization required by the employer contract or the termination of a physician from the existing organization with which the person is enrolled.

There is also an increasing trend for managed care organizations to allow members to use services outside of the established networks, with the member paying either all of the cost or the difference between what the HMO would have paid for the care and what was charged (American Association of Retired Persons Special Bulletin, 1996; Wagner, 1997). The type of contract that includes a stipulation that allows for flexibility in choosing a provider outside of the HMO is called a "point-of-service" plan. Such point-of-service opportunities provide some flexibility, allowing the members to retain some decision-making control.

Use of a Gatekeeper

Another strategy used by all managed care organizations is the use of "gatekeepers" to control entry into receiving health care. Enrolled members are required to choose a primary care physician, who is then responsible for managing the primary care needs of the member and making referrals to specialists as needed. The gatekeeper will determine if and when the member can see a specialist. It is the responsibility of the gatekeeper to ensure that all enrolled members get the right service at the right time and in the right place. A major goal of the use of a gatekeeper is to limit the use of emergency care and specialist care so that costs can be contained (Hurley, Freund, & Paul, 1993). The use of a gatekeeper curtails the choices for health care that the client can make. This aspect of the gatekeeper role has led, in recent years, to concern that it is more of a gate-*shutter* role (Bodenheimer & Grumbach, 1995). Consequently, recent legislative action at the state level has begun to address this issue. A number of states are passing legislation that provides greater decision making for the client, at least for emergency care (Miller, 1997).

Prospective Review

Another strategy used by the HMO is that of prospective review prior to use of a medical service. Prior to the physician or gatekeeper sending a patient to an outpatient service for diagnostic testing or to the acute-care hospital for treatment, the managed care organization must be notified and approval received. This process is commonly referred to as precertification for the need for care.

Kongstvedt (1997) lists several reasons why this process is used. The first is to notify the managed care organization that the need for acute-care services has arisen. This will alert the organization that plans for appropriate follow-up will need to be made. The second is to make sure that the care will be provided in the most appropriate setting. For example, it may be possible for the needed care to be provided on an outpatient basis, rather than an inpatient basis, as originally suggested by the physician. The third reason is to anticipate the financial cost of the service rather than be surprised when the bill is generated. All of these will assist the managed care organization to better control costs. When the organization approves the use of the requested service, the next strategy of managed care organizations can be implemented: utilization management.

Utilization Management

Utilization management is primarily geared toward services provided in either the subacute or tertiary care centers. At the time the health plan is notified of the need for medical services, the utilization management process is implemented.

The first step in this process is to assign a projected length of stay that will be required for the member to receive needed services. This is based on data provided by the primary care provider as to the diagnosis and projected treatment. In some plans, payment for services provided will cover only this designated period (Kongstvedt, 1997). This process has caused considerable concern among the public about managed care systems. Physicians are concerned that this process limits their ability to provide the required care. Many believe that additional variables, such as the severity of the illness, possible comorbidities, the extent of treatment needed, and environmental variables such as the person's socioeconomic status, are required to make an appropriate judgement as to the length of stay needed (Miller, 1997). Also, enrolled members need to have more information about how treatment decisions are made, in particular when a requested service is denied. Legislation at the state level is beginning to limit the power of the managed care organizations to make severity-of-treatment decisions without appropriate disclosure of the reasons for decisions that adversely affect their enrollees (Miller, 1997).

A feature common to many managed care organizations is the use of a utilization manager, who takes major responsibility for the coordination of care, thus preventing things from "falling between the cracks" (Shortell et al., 1996, p. 151). The utilization manager is employed by whoever is "at risk" for the cost of the treatment the enrolled member receives (Bodenheimer & Grumbach, 1995). Under a system in which the managed care plan and the hospital are part of the same organization, the plan will employ the utilization manager. If the contract places the risk for the payment on the hospital, it is wise for the hospital to employ its own utilization manager.

Nurses have become the most common health care provider to take on the utilization management function. Their role is to influence physician behavior so that treatment is provided in a cost-efficient manner. Their function is also to prevent the use of services that are deemed by the managed care organization to be unnecessary (Bodenheimer & Grumbach, 1995). The utilization manager will monitor the progress of all enrollees admitted to either a subacute or a tertiary hospital. This can be done by daily rounds at institutions where a significant number of the plan's members are hospitalized or by telephone contact with such institutions. Another responsibility of the utilization manager is to develop a discharge plan by anticipating the need for additional services such as long-term care, home care, or durable medical goods. The utilization manager must become an advocate both for the patient and the managed care organization.

Utilization management has become an integral component of managed care organizations. This system provides the information needed by the organization to control costs by unnecessary treatments or prolonged lengths of stay. It also, at times, sets up an adversarial relationship between the utilization management person and the physician (Kongstvedt, 1997). A well-developed procedure for managing such conflict is needed. Kongstvedt (1997) suggests that the utilization manager nurse should refer these conflict situations to the physician overseer of the utilization management program in the organization.

Communication Systems

Managed care organizations need to have a high level of communication between providers to truly coordinate care in a timely manner. Health care providers will have to become comfortable with computerized information systems that are used at the point of care; that is, at the patient's bedside in the hospital or at the physician's office (Elfrink, 1996). Also, because care is provided through a team approach, the need for increased trust among all team members is imperative. Team-building experiences will enhance this process.

Availability of Services

Care can only be coordinated if there is a sufficient number of services available to move a patient through the various levels of care provision, including primary, acute, restorative, and maintenance care services. If a "bottleneck" occurs at any point of the care continuum, health care dollars will be wasted while a patient is treated at a higher level of care than needed. The opposite can also happen. If a service is not available when needed, the person's condition could deteriorate, resulting in the requirement for a higher, more costly level of treatment than would have been needed earlier in the course of illness. A study done by Anders (1993) looked at problems in administrative delays in moving patients out of two acute-care hospitals. He found that the most frequent reason for delay in discharge was a lack of beds available in skilled nursing facilities, resulting in increased hospital costs.

Hand-Off Times

The times when coordination needs are at the highest are those that can be described as "hand-off" times. The admission of a patient to the hospital from a physician's office can produce a number of problems. The lack of timely and accurate information about the patient's treatment plan can prolong a hospital stay. If treatment orders do not arrive at the hospital along with the patient, time is lost in beginning the desired treatment plan. For example, in an oncology unit, it is important to have the orders for the chemotherapy regimen and current laboratory data to facilitate prompt treatment. If either of these are missing, the patient's acute-care stay will be longer than needed and excess expense will be incurred.

The discharge process is another critical time. The discharge plan must be in place in a timely manner so that a referral to a subacute setting, if needed, can be made and the bed secured for the patient. Home health care referrals, needs such as durable medical equipment, and appropriate teaching are also vital to moving the patient out of the acute-care environment as quickly as possible.

Other problems in the coordination of care can also occur. Each time a patient is seen by a new set of providers, redundant questioning can occur. This is both a nuisance to the patient and a waste of health provider efforts. This can result in a waste of resources, such as getting repeat lab values or other testing. Again, the use of coordinated information systems can help to solve this problem. Unfortunately, even in health care systems that use a computer database for managing information, this can be an issue. For example, if the acute-care hospital information system and the home health information system are not coordinated, there will be duplication of effort to establish a database for the patient newly discharged from the acute-care hospital to the home health system.

An important strategy for a managed care organization to develop is a mechanism with which to manage members with chronic health conditions. Ethridge (1991) has been able to document that the cost for providing services to members with chronic illness can be reduced by close management. Only through a tracking system will clients with minor health problems be managed so the problem does not become major. This need is an important reason why the field of nursing case management is rapidly expanding.

Health Promotion Strategies

The old paradigm of fee-for-service care focused on disease-state management in which the major portion of the health care dollar went to meeting needs caused by acute illness. This often necessitated the use of highly sophisticated resources in expensive tertiary settings. There was no provision, in the majority of health plans, for disease prevention programs. This emphasis must be reversed if the cost-effectiveness goal of managed care is to be achieved. Thus a major strategy of managed care should be an increased emphasis on disease prevention and health promotion. The cost-effectiveness goal of a managed care organization cannot be met without a strong emphasis on such programs. To do this, a health care system must be developed in which a significant portion of the health care dollar is spent on preventing disease and managing chronic illness before it reaches a high-intensity level.

However, there are several problems that need to be addressed to achieve this objective. The first relates to how the cost of preventive care can be demonstrated to provide cost effectiveness to the managed care organization. The cost of services to prevent complications stemming from chronic disease can be quite high. For example, a multisite study evaluated the effect of maintaining tight blood glucose control in insulin-dependent diabetics (Diabetes Control and Complications Trial Research Group, 1993). A significant reduction in complications was achieved when tight diabetic control was maintained; however, maintaining this tight control was very expensive. The cost savings gained from reducing amputations, blindness, and kidney failure, common outcomes of uncontrolled chronic diabetes, are not seen for many years. This demonstrates the principle that many prevention programs do not reap their benefits for a number of years. Thus they will not affect the current financial statement of a managed care organization.

Another problem in demonstrating financial return on health promotion activities is that members in managed care organizations have a pattern of moving from one managed care organization to another. Thus, the profit gained from preventive services may not come back to the organization that provided them. Marwick (1996) states that "managed care is a short term operation" (p. 768). One suggestion to remedy this problem is for all of the managed care organizations in an area to work together to provide prevention programs, thus sharing the cost burden. In this way, there would be more incentive for an HMO to spend money on prevention programs.

Another problem to overcome in developing strong health promotion programs is to find ways for managed care organizations to develop closer relationships with public health groups. The public health sector has had long experience in determining community health needs. By paying attention to the skills and knowledge developed by providers working in the public health sector, managed care organizations can learn much about the preventive aspect of health care. They also need to team up with social service agencies and community groups to identify the health needs that will provide the best return on the money invested. Shortell et al. (1996) suggest that managed care organizations will begin to incorporate public health strategies into their organizations because such strategies make economic sense. To do this, health care professionals working in the managed care sector need to learn new skills.

One new skill needed by health care professionals working in the managed care sector is community assessment techniques. These are needed to identify the appropriate prevention programs that will make an impact on the community (Primono, 1995). In the past, all too often, prevention programs were developed without a good understanding of community needs. An example of this is a mass mammogram screening program developed by the Indian Health Service to serve a Native American population (Steinhart, 1996). However, the rate of breast cancer in this population is only one half of that in the population as a whole (Trujillo, 1996). One must question if the money spent on this program would have been better spent on a diabetes education and management program, as the incidence of diabetes mellitus in this population is almost three times that of the general population (Trujillo, 1996). Managed care groups need to look at information such as this before determining how to spend the available health care dollars. Thus a major strategy needed for success in the managed care environment is population-based planning. New expertise is required in biostatistics and clinical epidemiology to interpret and use data more appropriately in the health planning process (Primono, 1995).

An important step in the health planning process is to conduct health screening of community residents and then plan health services based on the information obtained. The managed care agency should coordinate these activities with local health departments. An example of such coordination was a community health assessment done in Flagstaff, Arizona, in the summer of 1996 (Dean, 1996). This study was commissioned and funded by the local hospital, which is rapidly moving into a managed care configuration. A professional research group skilled in community assessment was brought in to conduct the actual survey. Strategies used to develop the database included the use of focus groups involving patients and community leaders, telephone surveys, and review of existing health studies. The information obtained identified several major community health problems, including domestic violence, access to health care services, access to prenatal care, and chronic and binge drinking (Dean, 1996). These problems, then, are target areas for the provision of coordinated health services by several agencies in the community, including the hospital, the local university, and other community-based service groups.

This approach uses the principles described by Shortell et al. (1996, p. 170) of an "outside-in" approach, in which one first investigates the health problems of the population. From these data, a target group is identified that is at risk for health problems. The individual patient is looked at last. This approach is contrary to the usual long-range planning strategies used by health care agencies in the past in which the organization first identified what services it would offer and then looked for patients requiring that service. Data obtained through this outside-in approach can also be used by health care organizations to enable them to determine what parts of the continuum of health care need to be developed. Such planning will lead to better integration of services in a community.

Some managed care organizations have already demonstrated the effectiveness of such strategies. The Group Health Cooperative of Puget Sound (Nudelman & Andrews, 1996) has placed a high emphasis on preventive activities. In one such endeavor, the organization targeted all of their members older than 65 years old for a flu immunization program. They were able to achieve a 70% immunization rate, which resulted in a dramatic drop in acute hospital admissions during the subsequent flu season. They also developed highly effective smoking cessation programs for high school and college students. Obviously, the cost-effectiveness of such a program will not be realized for many years. Another health promotion program developed by this group was a mammogram screening program, in which the group was able to screen its members at a far higher rate than the national average. Such programs provide great social benefit and will, at the same time, eventually reduce health care costs.

Another cost-effective program is provision of adequate prenatal care to all women. The cost-effectiveness of providing prenatal care for a woman to carry a pregnancy to full term has long been demonstrated. Figures reported in 1991 indicate that savings between $14,000 and $30,000 dollars can be obtained by avoiding one low birth weight infant (Office of Technology Assessment, 1991). Figures obtained from the Institute of Medicine (1988) indicate that there is a cost saving of $3.38 for every $1.00 spent in prenatal care. In examining these savings, one must consider that preventing a low-weight birth saves more than just the immediate intensive care expense. These premature babies often have health problems that remain with them for a lifetime, thus increasing the cost of health care for them over their life span.

Another area that needs to be addressed to reduce health care expenditures is that of domestic violence (Shortell et al., 1996). The cost of the injuries resulting from such violence is staggering. In the previously mentioned community health assessment done in Flagstaff, domestic violence was identified as one of the four major health problems (Dean, 1996). Thus, as managed care organizations consider health promotion programs, attention must be paid to more than just disease prevention programs. Rather, a comprehensive program of promoting health and preventing disease must include the means to address both social issues and medical problems.

Health education is another important element in managing the scarce health dollar resources. Some of the most common chronic health conditions found in the United States are hypertension, obesity, and diabetes, and these require intensive management. However, they are conditions that respond well to changes in lifestyle and thus are important areas to target for education. This education must encompass more than just providing information needed to make lifestyle changes; it must also include long-term support systems necessary for people to make these lifestyle changes that are needed to reduce health risks.

In summary, the focus of future health care systems must be to identify common health problems and find ways to prevent their escalation to the point where expensive tertiary care is needed. Health promotion and disease prevention need to become important strategies of managed care organizations. Nurses are well prepared to be leaders in this movement.

Quality Management

The development of quality management programs in managed care organizations is the final strategy required for their success that will be discussed. Provision of quality health care is becoming a topic of national debate because of the impact of negative public perceptions of managed care organizations. The rapid rise of the health maintenance organization (HMO) movement has spurred fears among the American public that more attention is paid to the cost of care than its quality. This concern has become so broad that a number of groups are forming to address this issue. At the federal level, a panel has been formed to study the effect of managed care organizations on providing quality health care. The issue of what percentage of the health dollar premium goes directly back to the consumer and how much is used to pay executive salaries is surfacing across the country. For example, employee unions are looking at how HMOs spend their dollars by reviewing what percentage goes directly into health care and what percentage is used for administrative costs. The demand by the public is to have a health care system in which quality care will be provided at a reasonable price. To understand such issues, one must first address the issue of quality.

What Is Quality Care?

Consensus on reaching a definition of quality has been difficult because of the number of confounding variables that are present in every patient situation. Some authors suggest that quality is related to the issues of effectiveness, efficiency, and appropriateness (Bower & Falk, 1996). Using this definition, quality is achieved when the appropriate service is provided in an efficient manner and the desired outcome is reached. Many health care organizations have used an industrial model for defining quality by focusing on the customer of the organization. Such a definition for quality would focus on meeting or exceeding the expectations of the customer. This has led to the development of a total quality management (TQM) program based on assessing economic outcomes.

Another definition states that quality is "the presence of socially acceptable desired attributes within the multifaceted holistic experience of being and doing" (Larrabee, 1996, p. 356). This definition goes beyond the industrial model of quality management to include the human experience in each situation. Some measurement of user satisfaction with the services provided is necessary. Most health care organizations use some type of customer satisfaction survey to collect these data. However, recent studies suggest that these data are not always provided to the clinical departments where improvement in service is needed (Nelson & Niederberger, 1990).

In a managed care organization, quality must be looked at from a variety of perspectives. In the past, quality assurance programs focused on retrospective analysis of what went wrong. Now, the focus is on how the process can be improved to provide for better customer outcomes. The current emphasis is to take a proactive rather than a reactive approach. Management of quality is now used even when no problems have been identified. The belief is that there is always room for improvement. With this focus, there has been a rapid growth in sophisticated programs for measurement of quality.

Quality Management Programs

The origins of the current quality management movement arose out of the work of Deming (1986) and Juran (1988). During the 1970s, Deming studied the rates of Japanese and American productivity and found that Japanese were superior. His study of the Japanese workplace indicated that the commitment to quality and listening to the customer were contributing factors to the predominance of Japan in the world marketplace. He brought back the idea of quality circles to the United States in which all persons involved in the production of a product met together to discuss means to improve the process. Deming's emphasis was on the collection, measurement, and analysis of data to improve production processes. This work fostered the development of total quality management (TQM) programs.

A newer movement in the management of quality is the continuous quality improvement (CQI) process, in which there is a shift of emphasis to identifying customer values. The focus of this movement is on accountability (Mitchell, 1994). Another new variation on the TQM/CQI process is the use of performance improvement (PI). In this program, the first step is to design new functions, processes, and services that are based on the mission of the organization. This strategy is of extreme importance to the managed care organization because of the paradigm shift that has occurred in setting priorities in health care. Applying old processes to the new environment will not work. Following the designing of the new processes, ways must be determined to measure their effectiveness. A systematic assessment must be done to determine if the desired goals and priorities are being met. Finally, improvements must be made to solve any problems identified in the assessment phase. A reiterative cycle is followed in which the processes used to achieve the desired quality goals are continually monitored and improved.

An example of a managed care system that has made a commitment to the TQM/CQI process is the Fairview Hospital Systems (Shortell et al., 1996). The overall goals identified for the organization include a focus on individual leadership, customers, process, people, and measurement. These goals represent the principles of the TQM/CQI concepts and identify areas for possible improvement projects.

To achieve the quality goals needed for successful managed care organizations, several subgoals need to be identified. These include the ability to reduce errors, meet standards set by outside reviewers, and measure provider-defined outcomes (Newell, 1996). Managed care organizations must also find ways to prevent clinical decisions from being made solely on the basis of cost. One strategy used by managed care organizations to accomplish this is to develop clinical practice guidelines that are agreed on by both the larger medical community and the internal medical community. These guidelines include a number of structured-care methodologies such as clinical (critical) pathways, standards of care, protocols, and algorithms (Cole, Lasker-Hertz, Grady, Clark, & Houston, 1996). If such standards are in place, both providers and the public will have an objective means of measuring the appropriateness of the care provided. At the same time, there must be a melding of what is effective care and what is within the reasonable financial means of the health care system. The old standard in the United States was to provide very high-tech care for the few. This must be altered to providing reasonable care for the masses. The use of common standards can be a means to make decisions on how to spend the health care dollar. Only when consensus can be reached about what constitutes effective care can there be a real measurement of quality in a managed care organization.

There is a great need to increase the emphasis on quality management, but there is still considerable debate on how best to do this. Newell (1996) suggests that traditional quality indicators such as morbidity and mortality are better suited to the old quality assurance process, a process that looked retrospectively at outcome measures. Effective quality management requires development of outcomes that are more customer focused. The use of such focused outcomes in studies has the potential to make a significant contribution to the achievement of the managed care goals of quality care. Nurses will need to become expert in designing and conducting such studies. Because the measurement of quality is of such importance to managed care organizations and thus to nurses, the entire next chapter will be devoted to discussing the specifics used in the evaluation of quality.

Conclusions

The provision of cost-effective quality health care requires that managed care organizations develop new operational strategies. Both the integration of services and coordination of care are necessary to meet the goal of cost effectiveness. As health care organizations increase in size and complexity to make these changes, their customer, the enrolled member, often has a difficult time in accessing needed health services. Nurses need to be in the forefront to help these customers deal with the complexities the larger organization brings. Consequently, coordination of client care has become a vital service.

Nurses have also demonstrated their importance to managed care organizations in fostering health promotion activities. Increases in both disease prevention and health promotion activities are necessary to reduce the need for expensive tertiary care. This is an area in which nurses excel. Finally, quality management strategies need to be emphasized as an important component of all health care organizations. The American public has begun to demand that financial considerations cannot be the only force driving the health care system.

New thinking is required to be successful in this environment; new approaches must be applied. As in any changing situation, it is difficult to learn new ways to function. For nurses to secure their rightful place in this new paradigm, an understanding of the underlying principles of how the managed care organizations function is necessary. This chapter has focused on making explicit the goals and strategies needed for success in today's health care world. Hopefully, it can serve as a looking-glass to turn the language of managed health care into a readable format.

References

American Association of Retired Persons Special Bulletin. (1996). *Special report: Managed care.* Washington, DC: AARP.

Anders, R. L. (1993). Administrative delays: Is there a difference between for-profit and non-profit hospitals? *Journal of Nursing Administration, 23*(11), 42-50.

Bodenheimer, T. S., & Grumbach, K. (1995). *Understanding health policy: A clinical approach.* Norwalk, CT: Appleton & Lange.

Bower, K. A., & Falk, C. D. (1996). Case management as a response to quality, cost, and access imperatives. In E. L. Cohen (Ed.), *Nurse case management in the 21st century* (pp. 161-167). St. Louis, MO: Mosby.

Cole, L., Lasker-Hertz, S., Grady, G., Clark, M., & Houston, S. (1996). Structured care methodologies. *Nursing Case Management, 1*(4), 160-172.

Dean, K. (1996). Health priorities. *Flagstaff Medical Center Corazon, 28*(5), 3.

Deming, W. E. (1986). *Out of crisis.* Cambridge, MA: MIT Center for Advanced Engineering Study.

Diabetes Control and Complications Trial Research Group. (1993). The effect of intensive treatment of diabetes on the development and progresion of long-term complications in insulin-dependent diabetes mellitus. *New England Journal of Medicine, 329*(14), 977-986.

Elfrink, V. (1996). Information technology: A tool for managing managed care. *Health Net, 10*(1), 2.

Ethridge, P. (1991). A nursing HMO: Carondelet St. Mary's experience. *Nursing Management, 22*(7), 22-27.

Gillies, R. R, Shortell, S. M., & Young, G. J. (1997). Best practices in managing organized delivery systems. *Hospital & Health Services Administration, 42*(3), 299-321.

Hurley, R. E., Freund, D. A., & Paul, J. E. (1993). *Managed care in Medicaid.* Ann Arbor, MI: Health Administration Press.

Institute of Medicine. (1988). *Prenatal care: Reaching mothers, reaching infants.* Washington, DC: National Academy Press.

Juran, J. M. (1988). *Juran on planning for quality.* New York: Free Press.

Kongstvedt, P. R. (1997). Managing basic medical-surgical utilization. In P. R. Kongstvedt (Ed.), *Essentials of managed health care* (2nd ed., pp. 199-224). Gaithersburg, MD: Aspen.

Kongstvedt, P. R., & Plocher, D. W. (1995). Integrated health care delivery systems. In P. R. Kongstvedt (Ed.), *Essentials of managed health care.* Gaithersburg, MD: Aspen.

Larrabee, J. H. (1996). Emerging model of quality. *Image: the Journal of Nursing Scholarship, 28*(4), 353-358.

Marwick, C. (1996). Effect of managed care felt in every medical field. *Journal of the American Medical Association, 276*(9), 672-676.

Menke, T. J. (1997). The effect of chain membership on hospital costs. *Health Services Research, 32*(2), 177-196.

Miller, T. E. (1997). Managed care regulation: In the laboratory of states. *Journal of the American Medical Association, 278*(13), 1102-1109.

Mitchell, M. (1994). How can we assure health care quality? In J. McCloskey & H. Grace (Eds.), *Current issues in nursing* (4th ed., pp. 287-294). St. Louis, MO: Mosby.

Nelson, C. W., & Niederberger, J. (1990). Patient satisfaction surveys: An opportunity for total quality improvement. *Hospital Health Service Administration, 35*, 409-427.

Newell, M. (1996). *Using nursing case management to improve health outcomes.* Gaithersburg, MD: Aspen.

Nudelman, P. M., & Andrews, L. M. (1996). The "value added" of not-for-profit health plans. *New England Journal of Medicine, 334*(16), 1057-1059.

Office of Technology Assessment, U.S. Congress. (1991). *Identifying health technologies that work: Searching for evidence* (Pub. No. OTA-H-608). Washington, DC: U.S. Government Printing Office.

Primono, J. (1995). Ensuring public health nursing in managed care: Partnerships for healthy communities. *Public Health Nursing, 12*(2), 69-71.

Shortell, S. M., Gillies, R. R., Anderson, D. A., Erickson, K. M., & Mitchell, J. B. (1996). *Remaking health care in America.* San Francisco: Jossey-Bass.

Steinhart, J. (1996). Program evaluation: Mammography at Shiprock, 1991-1994. *IHS Primary Care Provider, 21*(9), 119-125.

Trujillo, M. H. (1996). Looking to the future of the Indian Health Service. *IHS Primary Care Provider, 21*(12), 157-160.

Wagner, E. R. (1997). Types of managed care organizations. In P. R. Kongstvedt (Ed.), *Essentials of managed health care* (2nd ed., pp. 36-48). Gaithersburg, MD: Aspen.

Chapter

4

Nursing Involvement in Quality of Care Issues

Margaret M. Conger

> *It is imperative that the profession [nursing] measures and evaluates its work.*
>
> Blewitt and Jones (1996, p. 48)

Measurement of the quality of service provided is important to every business, including health care. However, the definition of quality and the means to measure it are under considerable debate. A superficial definition of quality is to do the right thing at the right time in the right way. Newell (1996) suggests that quality should be described as "meeting of fitness for use specification" (p. 157). In health care, this is measured by how closely the program meets the client-defined goals. Another way that quality can be measured in health care is how many "re-do's" are needed; that is, what additional treatment is needed because of inadequate or inappropriate treatment (Newell, 1996). Larrabee (1996) suggests that quality itself cannot be measured; only the desired attributes of quality are measurable. For many, this has come to mean that the outcomes resulting from the provision of care are what is to be measured. With such a variety of understandings of what quality is, it is little wonder that there is considerable debate about measurement methods.

In addition to quality being perceived as doing "the right thing," ethical considerations must also be considered. The issues of fairness and justice are important to a discussion of quality health care. What is fair to the consumer, the provider, the payer? Also, in the day of for-profit health care organizations, the economic expectations of the stockholder must also be met. No discussion of quality of care can be complete without considering its effect on each of these parties.

The ethical principles outlined in the Code for Nurses (American Nurses Association [ANA], 1985) make a strong case for the responsibility the nursing profession has for continually maintaining a high quality of care. How this quality of care will be measured is the question that needs to be explored. Newell (1996) suggests that the use of customer- (or patient-/client-)defined outcomes provides the most direct means to evaluate quality. There is, however, considerable debate over just how to do this. The nursing profession is actively exploring new ways to measure the quality of care provided by nurses. This chapter will discuss a number of techniques that have been used to assess the quality of health care provided.

The term used to describe the recipient of health care is changing. Traditionally, the person who sought care in a hospital or from a health care provider has been termed a patient. As health care has moved out into community settings, and as more health care providers embrace the concept that each person must take considerable responsibility for his or her own health, the term client is being used more frequently. In this chapter, the term client will be used to describe the recipient of health care in most cases; however, when the discussion is focused specifically on a situation that occurs within an acute-care hospital, the term patient will be used. For example, when talking about satisfaction levels with care provided, hospitals have traditionally used the term patient satisfaction rates. This practice will be followed in this book.

Traditional Quality Measurement Techniques

The classic patient care evaluation model developed by Donabedian (1966) includes ethical as well as economic principles to evaluate the quality of patient care. This model takes into consideration structure, process, and outcome variables. Structural variables include components such as the number and type of providers, practice regulations, characteristics of clients served, and payment mechanisms. Process is related to the actions of the provider and looks at issues such as how care is being managed. The focus of the evaluation is on determining whether procedures are carried out as planned. The outcomes that need to be examined include both quality and cost of care. In addition, the accessibility of the care to those requiring it is an important consideration. Typical outcome measures include how many resources are used in terms of cost, the adherence to established standards of care, and patient functional status following an episode of care. This model has been the basis for the origins of the quality assessment (QA) movement in health care. During the 1970s and 1980s, nurses in hospital settings were instrumental in developing quality assurance methodologies based on the Donabedian model.

Quality Assurance Methodologies

The quality assurance process has been traced to the work of Florence Nightingale during the Crimean War, when she evaluated the effect of nursing care on the soldiers' mortality rate (Decker & Sullivan, 1992; Huber, 1996). More recently, the evolution of quality assurance programs has been traced back to the development of nursing standards by the American Nurses Association (ANA) for use in evaluating nursing practice. These standards were often used by hospital nursing departments to evaluate the quality of care provided to patients. Reviews by the Joint Commission on Accreditation of Hospitals (JCAHO) spurred the rapid rise in quality assurance programs. The quality assurance process consisted of the development of predetermined standards of care, regular auditing of data to determine the percent compliance with those standards, and documented plans for the improvement of areas in which problems were found. A major flaw in this system was the focus on identifying problems without providing the resources or power for nurses to make system changes to solve identified problems. Also, the process focused on nursing care provided in a particular unit rather than looking at the issue from a multiunit perspective. The problems, however, often needed input from a variety of health care providers to improve care. Because of the limitations of the quality assurance process, new quality management programs have been derived.

Total Quality Management

The next progression in the measurement of quality was the development of total quality management (TQM) programs, which arose out of the work of Deming (1986). These programs stress the responsibility of the individual worker to be knowledgeable, accountable, and responsible (Arikian, 1991). They are based on the premise that when employees understand their jobs and their value to the organization, they will be motivated to make changes that will improve the product or service line in which they are engaged (Arikian, 1991). Such changes result in high-quality service and improved customer satisfaction.

The TQM process is used to evaluate the work done in an organization more globally than was found in the typical quality assurance process. The strategy of a TQM program is to empower individuals closest to providing a service to take responsibility for the outcomes achieved. To do this, the employees must have access to the tools needed to carry out the evaluation process. They must be given the authority to carry out whatever changes the evaluation process has shown to be needed to improve the quality of service. An emphasis of all TQM projects must be on streamlining work processes, with a goal of improved outcomes. The direction of the priorities must focus on defining, understanding, and meeting customer expectations, not employee goals.

Continuous Quality Improvement Process

Continuous quality improvement (CQI) is a further refinement of the quality management process. Many organizations now use a CQI process that provides for both the assessment of quality and a structure for making improvements similar to that used in the TQM process. CQI, however, adds a further dimension of a reiterative cycle in which the outcomes of one process are used to determine what changes will be made in the organization. The effects of these changes are then evaluated in the next cycle.

The CQI process is described by Siren and Laffel (1997) as a stepwise process in which the results of one cycle feed the questions of the next cycle. The steps in the CQI process are shown in Figure 4.1. The first step of the process is to identify customer needs through the analysis of data generated by patient satisfaction questionnaires, complaints, or the use of focus groups.

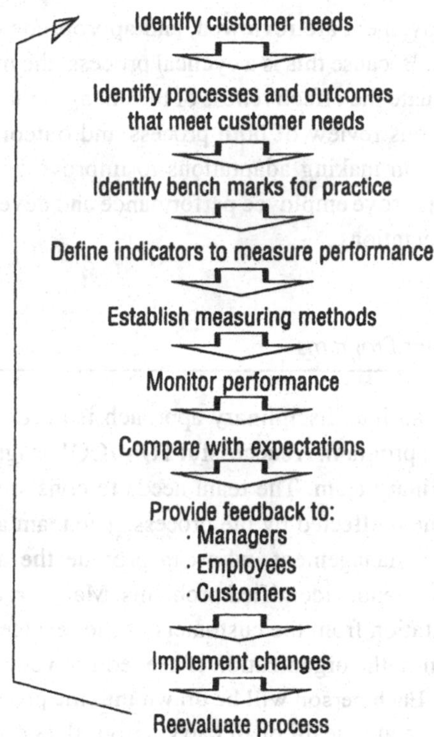

Figure 4.1 Continuous Quality Improvement Process
SOURCE: Adapted from Siren and Laffel (1997).

The next step is to identify the processes that will achieve the desired customer outcomes. In the health care setting, this focus is usually on processes used to treat a patient with an illness or to manage wellness activities. Next, data from other model organizations that are considered to be leaders in the field are gathered to form a basis for comparison. This process, in which one institution's performance is compared to a model organization, is called "benchmarking." Using data gathered in this process, outcomes are defined that can be used to measure the organization's performance. Methods to measure these outcomes are established, and the monitoring process is initiated.

Data obtained from the monitoring process are compared with the expected performance benchmarks, and the results are reported back to the organization's managers and employees, as well as to the customers. Areas identified for improvement are reviewed, and appropriate changes are made to correct problems. Because this is a cyclical process, the monitoring process will be used to evaluate the effectiveness of the changes made. The CQI cycle results in a continuous review of both process and outcomes measures and places an emphasis on making adaptations to improve quality. It functions well as a means to improve employee performance and develop processes that meet customer expectations.

Quality Management Programs

In health care, an interdisciplinary approach is needed for a successful quality management program. A successful TQM/CQI program requires input from a crossdisciplinary team. The team needs to consist of representatives from every department affected by the process. The team also needs to have representation from management, who can provide the authority to make necessary changes to handle identified problems. Many organizations also try to include representation from the customers of the service. The cooperation of every person within the organization is needed for a successful TQM/CQI process to proceed. Each person will be drawn into the process at some point, either as part of the actual team or in carrying out data collection and work improvement changes.

The outcomes used to measure quality are best developed by a team that crosses over traditional service areas. One department can no longer lay blame on another for problems that occur in the delivery of care (Gropper & Skarzynski, 1995). Most issues that affect customer needs are affected by several services and thus need the input from each of these services to achieve desired outcomes. For example, the management of a postoperative patient is dependent upon a multitude of services, such as the nursing care provided both in the postanesthesia unit and the medical/surgical unit. The anesthesia department is vital to the patient's care, both in the choice of the anesthesia used during surgery and in the management of postoperative pain. The physicians involved in directing the patient's care, as well as all of the allied health services such as dietary, pharmacy, and physical therapy, must also be part of the assessment process.

Tarlov et al. (1989) suggest a number of possible outcome measures that can be used by managed care organizations for assessing the quality of health care delivery. These are shown in Table 4.1. Clinical outcomes, such as a

TABLE 4.1 Outcome Measures for Assessing Quality of Care

- Clinical indicators
  - Clinical signs and symptoms
  - Laboratory data
- Functional status of client
  - Social
  - Mental
  - Role function
  - Health perception
  - Energy level
  - Pain level
  - Life satisfaction
- Customer satisfaction with care
  - Access to care
  - Convenience of care
  - Adequacy of financial coverage

decrease in the signs or symptoms of a disease process or laboratory values that the client will achieve at a specified time, need to be established and measured for a specific health issue. The functional status that a client should achieve at the specified end point of care should also be determined. This includes measures of social, mental, and role status attained, including such criteria as the person's health perception, energy level, pain level, and life satisfaction. Finally, all managed care organizations need to look at issues of customer satisfaction with care. These should include satisfaction with access to care, the convenience of the care, and adequacy of financial coverage provided by the health plan.

Powell (1996) points out that although the emphasis of a TQM/CQI program is to achieve a high level of performance throughout the organization, there is still a need to react to crisis and to monitor actual or potential problems. Thus, the TQM/CQI process must also include some of the elements of the former quality assurance programs. This, however, cannot be where the emphasis of the program is placed. There must be a commitment to continually look for ways to improve programs even when no problems are found.

Because a model such as the TQM/CQI process is strongly imbedded in an industrial model of quality, some nursing leaders suggest that a broader view of quality management is required to measure the effectiveness of nursing care (Larrabee, 1996). The remainder of this chapter will explore ways in which outcomes of nursing care can be evaluated.

Specific Quality Indicators

Traditional Indicators

Traditional indicators for measuring quality of health care have been mortality, morbidity, and length of stay (LOS) rates. However, there is some question about the relevance of these to nursing care. Mortality is more closely related to the patient's condition than to specific nursing interventions. Client characteristics such as age, severity of illness, and extent of comorbidities have a closer correlation with mortality rates (Newell, 1996). One study (Aiken, Smith, & Lake, 1994) makes a case for the quality of nursing care as a factor in improving mortality rates in a Medicare population. This study found that characteristics of nursing practice such as autonomy and open communication channels with physicians and other health care providers were the significant factors in the improved mortality rates in the hospitals surveyed.

Morbidity, the rate at which unforeseen events follow from the primary treatment, is also difficult to relate specifically to the quality of nursing care. Some aspects of morbidity, such as hospital-acquired infections, can have a direct relationship to nursing care: however, the complexity of conditions that lead to increased morbidity makes it difficult to ascribe changes in the morbidity rate to the quality of nursing care.

Likewise, the LOS of a patient is often an event in which nursing has little control. Physician preferences, patient and family capabilities, and other health provider availabilities probably have more effect on LOS than do nursing interventions. Also, Reiley and Howard (1995) found that the most accurate predictor of LOS in elderly people was the client's functional status, rather than provider action. Thus the use of these traditional indicators as measures of quality of nursing care must be questioned. New indicators that are more nurse sensitive are needed.

Nurse-Sensitive Indicators

A variety of nurse-sensitive indicators have been proposed for use in evaluating the quality of nursing care provided. Some of these are related to the traditional indicators of mortality and morbidity already discussed; many of them focus on entirely new areas. A list of these indicators is shown in Table

TABLE 4.2 Nurse-Sensitive Quality Indicators

- Morbidity
    - Infection rates related to:
        - Use of universal precautions
        - Management of intravenous catheters
        - Management of urinary catheters
        - Management of wound dressings
- Risk management issues
    - Patient fall rates
    - Pressure ulcer development
    - Medication error rates
- Patient satisfaction
- Provider satisfaction
- Control of symptoms
- Patient attributes
    - Psychosocial status
    - Ability to perform
        - Self-care activities
        - Instrumental activities of daily living
- Caregiver burden

4.2. Although many of the factors related to morbidity lie outside the control of nursing, infection rates for hospitalized patients are definitely nurse sensitive. Prevention of infection has historically been in the province of nursing (Bonadonna & Johnson, 1992). Practices related to the use of universal precautions, intravenous and urinary catheter management, and dressings techniques are directly controlled by nurses; thus, infection-control-related indicators have long been a part of quality assessments in the hospital setting. Other indicators over which nursing has considerable control that are used to measure quality include risk management perspectives, such as rates of patient falls, development of pressure ulcers, and medication errors. However, morbidity rates as a whole are affected by the actions of multiple groups of care providers and thus do not effectively reflect nursing interventions.

Patient and provider satisfaction rates are other indicators often used to measure quality. Virtually all hospitals collect data on patient satisfaction; however, the issues associated with such questionnaires often have little to do with nursing care. Lehr and Strosberg (1991) suggest that the results of these questionnaires often have little effect on influencing quality because the ability of patients to define and evaluate quality is questioned. Data obtained from provider satisfaction studies are even less valued. Few institutions have included regular evaluation of employee satisfaction as part of a quality management program. This practice may be shortsighted. Nakota and Saylor (1994) suggest that if staff nurses are satisfied with their role, they will be more productive and the institution will see improved patient outcomes. Employee satisfaction may well be an area that health care institutions need to include in quality improvement programs.

The quality of life of the client is another important area that can reflect on the effectiveness of nursing care. An important contributor to quality of life is the degree of control the person has over symptom management (Papenhausen, 1996). Nurses are very instrumental in working with clients, both to learn techniques needed for symptom management and to obtain the necessary equipment for such management.

A number of other nurse-sensitive indicators have been proposed for use in evaluating the quality of nursing care provided. The client's psychosocial status is an area for evaluation. One measure of this is his or her stress level at a specified point in care (Brooten & Nalor, 1995). This may be related to the client's quality of life. Social satisfaction, the ability to participate in social activities with family and friends, is an example of such an indicator. However, social satisfaction is affected by multiple factors. Hyland (1992) suggests that individual differences in mood, cognitive styles, or coping styles have a strong influence on perceived quality of life, all attributes of personality that the nurse has no control over. A number of assessment instruments have been developed to assess a person's psychosocial status. For example, the Mini Mental Status Exam can be used to determine a person's mental state (Folstein, Folstein, & McHugh, 1975).

The ability of a person to carry out the self-care activities of grooming, dressing, bathing, and ambulation is another area that can be used to reflect quality-of-nursing concerns. Other indicators include instrumental activities of daily living such as household activities and shopping. These can be measured with a tool such as the Functional Status Questionnaire (Jette, Davies, & Cleary, 1986). Again, the nurse can have a great impact on assisting clients and families in finding ways to meet these important needs.

Another area for possible evaluation of the quality of nursing care is the burden of caregiving in providing for client needs (Girouard, 1996). Nurses are important in helping families manage the demands of caring for a chronically or terminally ill family member. A tool such as the Caregiver Strain Index (Robinson, 1983) can be used to assess the level of the burden of care.

Caregiver burden has been shown to be inversely related to the client's functional status. Measurement of the care burden is important because, when it is high, the family will often need the assistance of a nurse to help sort through care options ranging from increased home health assistance to placement of the client in a long-term care facility (Gold, Reis, Markiewicz, & Andres, 1995).

With nursing moving from a largely hospital-based practice into a wide variety of community settings, there is increasing need to broaden the base of nurse-sensitive outcome indicators. The challenge now is to select those measures that reflect the goals of the environment in which nursing care is delivered.

Risk Management

Risk management has long been an area included in quality of care considerations. Powell (1996) describes it as a process in which major risk areas are identified and interventions are planned and executed that enhance patient safety and prevent problems before they occur. Unfortunately, in many organizations, the preventive process does not occur, and the risk management department then functions as "damage control" (Kongstvedt, 1993, p. 166). Because the prevention of loss is so important to obtaining the quality and cost goals of managed care organizations, every TQM/CQI program must include strategies to identify possible risk situations and manage patient care to reduce that risk.

The ANA (1996) recently identified quality standards for acute-care hospitals that link nursing actions and patient outcomes. Measurement of nosocomial infection rates related to urinary tract infections is one of the indicators. The recommendation for this measurement is to calculate the rate per 1000 patient care days at which patients develop a urinary tract infection in the first 72 hr of the hospital stay. For example, if an institution has 30 urinary tract infections among patients during their first 72 hours of hospitalization during a month in which 1000 patient days occurred, the infection rate would be 3%.

Guidelines for measuring patient injury rates have also been established (ANA, 1996). The rate of patient falls that result in injury during the course of the hospital stay per 1000 patient days is calculated. The guidelines also recommend that an analysis be done of the relationship between nursing assessments to identify patients at high risk for a fall and the number of patients who actually sustain an injury as the result of a fall. Such a study could demonstrate the effectiveness of programs that preidentify patients at high risk for falls and could institute preventive measures.

A third area of risk management that affects nursing is the maintenance of skin integrity (ANA, 1996). This measures the rate at which patients develop a Grade II or higher pressure ulcer later than 72 hours following admission to the hospital. Again, a secondary analysis of the relationship between a nursing assessment to identify patients at high risk for pressure ulcer development and those who actually develop a Grade II or higher pressure ulcer is recommended.

Other quality measures that reflect nursing concerns identified by the ANA Safety and Quality Initiative Task Force (ANA, 1996) include patient satisfaction rates with nursing care, pain management, and educational information. This task force also recommends that quality management programs include analysis of nurse satisfaction rates, skill mix, and total hours of nursing care provided per patient day. These all appear to indirectly affect risk management issues.

Measurement of Outcomes

One of the problems in the past in developing indicators that reflect nursing interventions has been an "all or nothing" approach (Johnson & Mass, 1997). Nurses have long identified desired outcomes of care such as "will walk 25 feet prior to discharge" or "will safely administer insulin prior to discharge." In measuring such outcomes, the client either did or did not meet them. Measurement based on a continuum will provide greater flexibility in the interpretation of outcome data; when a client partially meets an outcome, some credit is given (Johnson & Maas, 1997). The Nursing Outcome Classification System, as developed by Johnson and Maas, consists of 190 outcomes of nursing interventions that contain definitions, indicators, and measurement scales that can be used with either individual clients or with families as caregivers. For each outcome, an appropriate 5-point scale has been developed to rate the client's progress. These scales vary based on the nature of the outcome. For example, the outcome that measures mobility level consists of 5 levels of function:

Dependent, does not participate = 1
Requires assistive person and device = 2
Requires assistive person = 3
Independent with assistive device = 4
Completely independent = 5 (Johnson & Maas, 1997, p. 203)

The outcome for coping ability uses a different 5-point rating scale, consisting of the following statements:

Never demonstrated = 1
Rarely demonstrated = 2
Sometimes demonstrated = 3
Often demonstrated = 4
Consistently demonstrated = 5 (p. 136)

Data obtained from these scales can be used both to measure individual client behavior and as aggregate data to develop realistic standards of care. It can also be used to identify realistic target goals for individual clients rather than setting the same standard for each client with a similar diagnosis. When unrealistic expectations are established for a particular client, resources will be wasted trying to reach an unobtainable goal (Johnson & Maas, 1997).

Resource Utilization

In the era of managed care, resource utilization is another measure used by organizations to evaluate the quality of services provided. Resource utilization includes a variety of parameters, such as use of supplies, equipment, or services, provided by various departments in the organization. Use of expensive treatment areas, such as emergency departments, operating rooms, or intensive care units, must also be monitored because their use has a great impact on the cost of care. Because personnel costs are a large part of any health care organization, they must be closely monitored. The skill mix used to care for patients has received considerable attention. It is important to use the most cost-effective provider able to safely manage the complexity of the required care. Indicators developed by the ANA Nursing Safety and Quality Initiative (ANA, 1996) that track the ratio of RNs both to assistive nursing personnel and to the total hours of patient care per day are useful in measuring the type and amount of nursing resources used. A health care organization can only reach its goals when its clients receive high-quality care in a resource-efficient manner.

Ethical Principles

Ethical principles are the foundation upon which nursing practice is based. The Preamble to the Code for Nurses (ANA, 1985) states that nurses "make a moral commitment to uphold the values and special moral obligations expressed in their code" (p. i). The decisions made by nurses concerning client care issues must be based on universal moral principles. Thus, when discussing the quality of care received by recipients of nursing care, ethical issues must be considered.

Larrabee (1996) has developed a model that demonstrates a relationship between quality of care and four ethical principles: beneficence, value, justice, and prudence. These principles have an impact on all nursing interactions. In the top portion of Figure 4.2, the relationship between ethical principles and nursing interventions is shown. These principles surround all nursing interventions and influence the way in which nursing is provided. They also influence the outcomes resulting from nursing care.

Beneficence is defined in this model as the "intention, capacity, and means for doing good" (Larrabee, 1996, p. 355). Another definition (Fromer, 1981) defines beneficence as the "obligation or duty to promote good, to further a person's legitimate interests, and to actively prevent or remove harm" (p. 317). Benefits to the client occur as an outcome of beneficence. The good referred to as an outcome of beneficence is not only the goal of the individual but of the group as well. This arises out of Aristotle's belief that a higher value is placed on group good because of the belief that the individual will suffer if the group or society suffers. Thus, quality cannot be measured only by individual goal achievement; group goal achievement must also be part of the measurement. Value is important to this model because the very use of the word *good* infers that a value is placed on the goals achieved. Value implies that something is intrinsically worthwhile.

Justice is also included in this model for evaluating quality of care. Larrabee (1996) argues that justice is important to quality measurement because of its impact on health care economics. Justice is defined as the maintenance of what is right and fair. A justice perspective suggests that

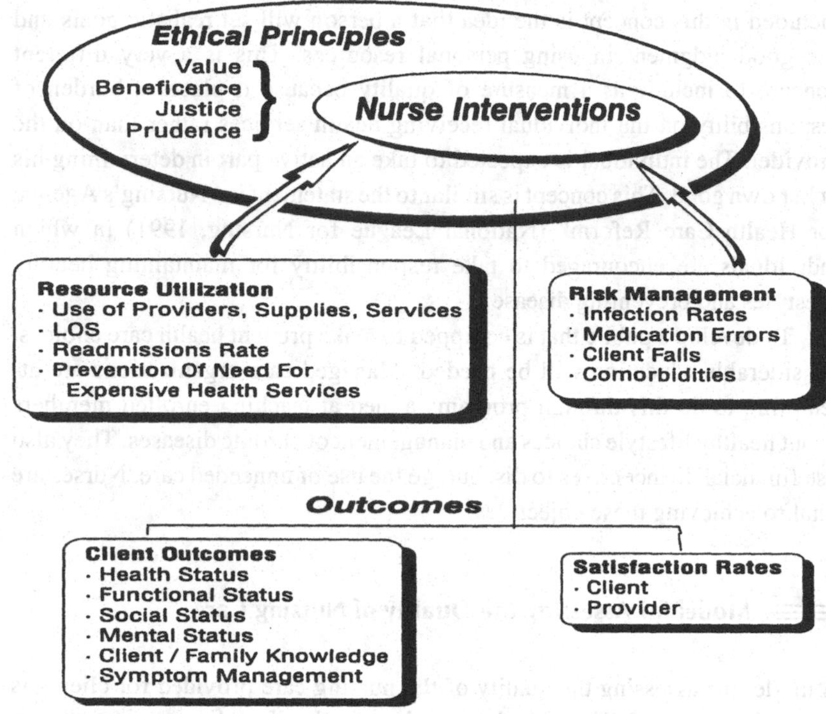

Figure 4.2 Model for Nursing Quality Assessment

individuals take only their fair share of the common resources based on their contribution to the common resources, a principle imbedded in the idea of distributive justice. Issues that must be addressed when considering quality from a justice perspective include the need to discuss questions such as who should receive services and who should pay for these services, particularly for the poor. Because health care costs are largely borne by the group as a whole rather than by the individual, decisions about how resources will be used become a public affair. Consequently, there is a need to develop quality measures that reflect the good of the community as well as the individual. A part of this analysis must be consideration of access to care, including the availability of services to the persons who need them.

The final component of this model for measuring quality of care is the concept of prudence. Contained within this concept is the idea of self-sufficiency and appropriate use of resources to achieve one's own goals. Also included in this concept is the idea that a person will set realistic goals and use good judgment in using personal resources. This is a very different concept to include as a measure of quality because it places a burden of responsibility on the individual receiving health services rather than on the provider. The individual is expected to take an active part in determining his or her own good. This concept is similar to the statement in "Nursing's Agenda for Health Care Reform" (National League for Nursing, 1991) in which individuals are encouraged to take responsibility for maintaining healthy lifestyles and preventing disease.

To develop a public that is equipped to make prudent health care choices, considerable education will be needed. Managed care organizations are attempting to do this through programs aimed at teaching enrolled members about healthy lifestyle choices and management of chronic diseases. They also use financial disincentives to discourage the use of unneeded care. Nurses are vital to achieving these objectives.

Model for Assessing the Quality of Nursing Care

A model for assessing the quality of the nursing care provided for clients is shown in Figure 4.2. The ethical principles of value, beneficence, justice, and prudence are shown surrounding all nursing interventions. Resource utilization both affects nursing interventions and is affected by them. Factors included in the evaluation of resource utilization include the use of providers, supplies, and services. Other factors included are the length of stay and readmission rates. Both of these are a direct reflection of services provided. An important element in reducing resource utilization is the prevention, by appropriate client management, of the need for expensive services. Risk management issues such as infection rates, medication errors, and client falls are all integrally tied to nursing interventions. These risk situations are minimized when nursing quality is high.

The quality of nursing care can be evaluated by the outcomes achieved, including both client outcomes and satisfaction rates. Outcomes that need to be assessed are the client's health and the client's functional, social, and mental status at the end of the episode of care. The knowledge level of the client and family in relationship to self-care abilities is also important to assess. Finally, the ability of the client to manage the symptoms inherent in a chronic health condition should be measured. Client satisfaction with care and provider satisfaction with working conditions are also important outcome outcomes to be assessed.

A model such as this provides a broader perspective of quality than do traditional methods that focus only on outcomes such as mortality, morbidity, and risk management issues. The indicators suggested here more closely reflect areas that the nurse has considerable ability to affect. They also provide a means to demonstrate the value that nursing care has for affecting the quality of care provided by a health care organization.

Measurement of Cost-Effectiveness

In any model for measuring quality in a managed care setting, cost must be a consideration. As early as 1974, Fuchs, a health care economist, realized that health care resources were scarce and that choices would have to be made between the competing needs for these resources. Recognition of the scarcity of resources is even more apparent today. Money spent on providing health care means that some other service will have to be decreased. Thus, appropriate use of resources must be determined based on a balance between the cost of the resource used and the benefit gained by the recipients of the care. Determining benefit is difficult because people place varying degrees of importance on how much health care is really desired. It is not uncommon for a person to state that he or she desires to remain healthy and yet practice behaviors such as smoking, overeating, or not exercising that decrease his or her health outcomes. Thus, when evaluating health and use of resources, the issues are not clear.

Another problem in evaluating the use of health care resources is the perspective that one brings to any situation. Fuchs (1974) describes three possible perspectives that can be taken. The first is a romantic perspective, in which the person does not understand the ramifications of the scarcity of resources. This lack of understanding leads to failure to make choices about how resources will be used. Consequently, no constraints are used and the result is continually escalating health care costs.

The second perspective is described as monotechnic, in which a person believes that the most advanced technological approach to a health problem is best. With this belief, the cost of the strategy is not considered, and alternative therapies that may be less resource expensive are not considered. The person fails to see that health problems can be managed by more than one means. Persons coming from both the romantic and the monotechnic perspective view quality as providing the best of available technology without consideration of cost.

An economic perspective is the third possible way of viewing the use of health care resources. A person with this perspective recognizes that resources are scarce and there are multiple competing demands for their use. Decisions about the allocation of health care resources must be made by evaluating the benefits that will be gained (Larrabee, 1996). This economic perspective is the basis for the cost-benefit process used in evaluating health care resource allocation.

Use of Health Care Resources

Resources must be used wisely to achieve the goal of cost-effective health care. Concern about health care finances is a new consideration for most nurses because the cost of nursing care has long been buried in the room charge in the acute-care hospital. In the past, little attention was paid to the amount of nursing resources required for any one patient. However, nursing staff makes up a large portion of the employees of any hospital, and thus increased scrutiny is now placed on how nurses are used to provide patient care.

A current practice in many hospitals has been to decrease the ratio of nurses to patients in an effort to reduce cost. This has been done with very little study to determine its effectiveness. One of the few studies done to look at this issue showed that when the labor efficiency ratio reached 120% (understaffing) the rate of complications rose by 30% and the mean length of stay increased by 3.5 days (Behner, Fogg, Fournier, Frankenbach, & Robertson, 1992). Managed care organizations need to look very closely at both patient and financial outcomes prior to reducing nursing staffing ratios.

McCormick (1986) suggests that new ways to demonstrate the effect of nursing on managing hospital costs must be found if nursing is going to survive as a profession. Nursing can affect the achievement of positive financial outcomes in several ways. One strategy is for nurses to work with clients and families to help them spend the available health care dollars in a fiscally sound manner. The nurse can guide clients to select appropriate resources, keeping in mind an economic perspective. This needs to occur in both community settings and hospital settings.

In the acute-care setting, the nurse can have a positive impact on length of stay by planning for discharge at the time of admission (Manss, 1993). Increasing the availability of nurses to manage the patient during the hospitalization period is another important way in which hospital costs can be reduced. Nurses working in the role of case manager have demonstrated that coordinated management of client care saves the health care system money by reducing both delays in provision of services and duplication of services. Another way that nurses can demonstrate their fiscal relevance is through the management of clients following discharge from a hospital. If, through nurse follow-up, a decrease in hospital readmission rates can be demonstrated, significant savings will be achieved.

Measurement of Cost Savings

In addition to the previously mentioned strategies for effecting health care cost savings, other measures also need to be developed. One such method is a cost-benefit analysis. This is a technique that compares the costs spent on preventive activities that result in savings from not using more expensive treatment options with the cost of these expensive treatments. It can also be used to demonstrate cost savings by using a less costly service such as home care instead of acute hospital care. The analysis includes a statement of the problems the client presented with, the plan of care used, the cost of this plan of care, and the projected costs if an alternate, more expensive care provision is made (Mullahy, 1995).

A cost benefit analysis is done by calculating all of the costs of services that are currently being provided to a client; it includes the costs of providers, supplies, and any institutional costs. This will give a total picture of what is being expended to provide for present client services. An estimate must then be done to calculate the savings achieved if changes are made so that the present level of service is no longer needed. The difference between continuing the service at the present level and changing the provided service to a less costly level is determined. This figure represents the net savings that can be achieved. Calculations of this type have not traditionally been done when determining health care expenditures. However, as the movement into managed care increases, such calculations are becoming essential.

Clinical Example

A cost-benefit analysis can be illustrated through the use of a case study. An elderly woman was admitted to an acute-care hospital with advanced liver failure and renal insufficiency. Her social history revealed that she lived alone but had a son who was visiting at the time of the acute exacerbation of her illness. She was eligible for health care coverage under Medicare and also had supplemental insurance that would pay for acute-care hospitalization but would not cover skilled nursing care.

It was quickly established following admission that no aggressive treatment for this patient was appropriate. The nurse case manager (NCM) met with the patient and her son and explained the terminal nature of the present illness. It was stressed that the treatment planned was to provide comfort only. The NCM then worked with the son and some close friends of the patient to make arrangements for discharge to home with assistance from the home nursing service, physical therapy, nursing aides, and a meals on wheels program.

The woman returned to her home with the health services arranged and had 6 fairly comfortable days. On the 7th day, she experienced an intracranial bleed and returned to the hospital. She exhibited gross neurological deficits that would prevent her from returning home with the level of services previously provided. She had no insurance coverage to pay for long-term care, but her insurance would pay for hospice care. The NCM negotiated with the insurance company to apply her hospice benefits to cover the cost of a stay in an extended-care facility. With this negotiation achieved, the patient was transferred to the extended-care facility and died there 2 weeks later.

In calculating the cost-benefit analysis for this woman's care, the actual expenses must be compared with what might potentially have been spent had skilled management of this patient not occurred. The cost savings to the hospital were 20 days of potential hospitalization, 6 of which would have occurred following the first admission and 14 following the second admission. At a hospitalization rate of $1,256.00 per day, this would amount to over $25,000 for the hospital room alone. Added to this amount would be the cost of supplies and services used.

The cost of the services provided at the lesser intensity of care were also calculated. This included the cost of three home health nurse visits, daily nursing aid care for 4 hours per day, two physical therapy visits, and rental of a hospital bed for the 6 days that the patient was at home. In addition, the cost

TABLE 4.3 Cost-Benefit Analysis

Costs Based on Plan Developed by Nurse Case Manager		*Charges Avoided by Plan Developed by Nurse Case Manager*	
Home services			
Home health nurse:		Acute care hospital	
3 visits @ $55.00/visit	= $ 165.00	days–20 @ $1,256/day	= $25,120.00
Physical therapist:			
2 visits @ 65.00/visit	= 130.00		
Home health aid:	= 180.00		
6 visits @ 30.00/visit			
Hospital bed: 6 days	= 10.00		
Delivery fee	= 20.00		
Skilled nursing facility: 14 days	2,000.00		
Total expenses	$ 2,505.00	Projected expenses	$25,120.00
Net savings	$22,615.00		

of a skilled nursing facility for 14 days was added to the calculation. The total cost for the lesser intensity of care came to $2,505.00. The calculations for this analysis are shown in Table 4.3. The net savings gained by appropriate patient management was $22,615.00.

In addition to the financial savings realized by successful case management in this situation, the human costs must also be considered. The 6 days that this woman spent at home with her family and friends nearby were invaluable to all. With the additional support services provided, the family was able to manage her care and allow her to remain in her home until she was at a point where she was no longer aware of her surroundings. The human gain is impossible to calculate in financial terms. This example illustrates how quality care and cost-effective goals can be met simultaneously. Such care should be the goal of all health care providers.

Conclusions

Outcome measures that reflect the quality of care provided by a health care organization are vital to the success of that organization. Health care consumers are becoming more educated in comparing available health care organizations to determine which gives the best value. The data generated from quality assessments will be used by these consumers to make decisions as to where they can obtain the best value for their health care dollars. The organization that can best demonstrate quality outcomes will be the one most likely to succeed in the future.

The measurement of quality of care is a complex issue in any organization. The old quality measures that included mortality, morbidity, and risk management issues are no longer sufficient. Nursing, in particular, must develop new ways to assess its effectiveness to survive in this new world. Because nurses are increasingly working in community settings, new indicators are needed to address the concerns that this type of care brings. In this chapter, a number of such indicators have been discussed. The use of nurse-sensitive indicators such as efficient resource utilization, positive client health outcomes, and ethically appropriate care is also important to establish the place of nursing in the new health care paradigm.

References

Aiken, L. H., Smith, H. L., & Lake, E. (1994). Lower medicare mortality among a set of hospitals known for good nursing care. *Medical Care, 32*(8), 771-787.

American Nurses Association. (1985). *Code for nurses with interpretive statements.* Washington, DC: Author.

American Nurses Association. (1996). *Nursing quality indicators for acute care settings.* Retrieved September 4, 1998, from the World Wide Web: http://www.nursingworld.org/readroom/fssafety.htm

Arikian, V. L. (1991). Total quality management: Applications to nursing service. *Journal of Nursing Administration, 21*(6), 46-50.

Behner, K. G., Fogg, L. F., Fournier, L. C., Frankenbach, J. T., & Robertson, S. B. (1992). Nursing resource management: Analyzing the relationship between costs and quality in staffing decisions. In M. Brown (Ed.), *Nursing management: Issues and ideas* (pp. 17-25). Gaithersburg, MD: Aspen.

Blewitt, D. K., & Jones, K. R. (1996). Using elements of the nursing minimum data set for determining outcomes. *Journal of Nursing Administration, 26*(6), 48-56.

Bonadonna, I. A., & Johnson, J. U. (1992). Integrating infection control into a nursing quality program. *Journal of Nursing Care Quality, 6*(4), 75-80.

Brooten, D., & Naylor, M. D. (1995). Nurses' effect on changing patient outcomes. *Image: the Journal of Nursing Scholarship, 27*(2), 95-99.

Decker, P. J., & Sullivan, E. J. (1992). *Nursing administration.* Norwalk, CT: Appleton & Lange.

Deming, W. E. (1986). *Out of crisis.* Cambridge, MA: MIT Center for Advanced Engineering Study.

Donabedian, A. (1966). Evaluating the quality of health care. *Millbank Quarterly, 44*, 166-206.

Folstein, M. F., Folstein, S. E., & McHugh, P. R. (1975). Mini-mental state: A practical method for grading the cognitive state of patients for clinicians. *Journal of Psychiatric Research, 12*, 189-198.

Fromer, M. J. (1981). *Ethical issues in health care*. St. Louis, MO: Mosby.

Fuchs, V. R. (1974). *Who shall live? Health, Economics, and Social Choice*. New York: Basic Books.

Girouard, S. A. (1996). Evaluating advanced nursing practice. In A. B. Hamric, J. A. Spross, & C. M. Hanson (Eds.), *Advanced nursing practice: An integrative approach* (pp. 567-600). Philadelphia: Saunders.

Gold, D. P., Reis, M. F., Markiewicz, D., & Andres, D. (1995). When home caregiving ends: A longitudinal study of outcomes for caregivers of relatives with dementia. *Journal of American Geriatrics Society, 43*(1), 10-16.

Gropper, E. L., & Skarzynski, J. J. (1995). Integrating quality assessment and improvement. *Nursing Management, 26*(3), 22-23.

Huber, D. (1996). *Leadership and nursing care management*. Philadelphia: Saunders.

Hyland, M. E. (1992). A reformulation of quality of life for medical science. *Quality of Life Research, 1*, 276-272.

Jette, A. M., Davies, A. R., & Cleary, P. D. (1986). The functional status questionnaire: Reliability and validity when used in primary care. *Journal of General Internal Medicine*, (1), 143-149.

Johnson, M., & Maas, M. (1997). *Nursing outcomes classification*. St. Louis, MO: Mosby.

Kongstvedt, P. R. (1993). *The managed health care handbook*. Gaithersburg, MD: Aspen.

Larrabee, J. H. (1996). Emerging model of quality. *Image: the Journal of Nursing Scholarship, 28*(4), 353-358.

Lehr, H., & Strosberg, M. (1991). Quality improvement in health care: Is the patient still left out? *Quality Review Bulletin, 17*, 326-329.

Manss, V. V. (1993). Influencing the rising costs of health care: A staff nurse's perspective. *Nursing Economics, 11*(2), 83-86.

McCormick, B. (1986, November 5). What's the cost of nursing care? *Hospitals, 60*(21), 48-52.

Mullahy, C. M. (1995). *The case manager's handbook*. Gaithersburg, MD: Aspen.

Nakota, J. A., & Saylor, C. S. (1994). Management style and staff nurse satisfaction in a changing environment. *Nursing Administration Quarterly, 18*(3), 51-57.

National League for Nursing. (1991). *Nursing's agenda for health care reform*. New York: Author.

Newell, M. (1996). *Using nursing case management to improve health outcomes*. Gaithersburg, MD: Aspen.

Papenhausen, J. L. (1996). Discovering and achieving client outcomes. In E. L. Cohen (Ed.), *Nurse case management in the 21st century* (pp. 257-268). St. Louis, MO: Mosby.

Powell, S. K. (1996). *Nursing case management: A practical guide to success in managed care*. Philadelphia: Lippincott-Raven.

Reiley, P., & Howard, E. (1995). Predicting hospital length of stay in elderly patients with congestive heart failure. *Nursing Economics, 13*(4), 210-216.

Robinson, B. C. (1983). Validation of a caregiver strain index. *Journal of Gerontology, 38*(3), 344-348.

Siren, P. B., & Laffel, G. L. (1997). Quality management in managed care. In P. R. Kongstvedt (Ed.), *Essentials of managed health care* (2nd ed., pp. 274-298). Gaithersburg, MD: Aspen.

Tarlov, A., Ware, J. E., Greenfield, S., Nelson, E. C., Perrin, E., & Zubkoff, M. (1989). The medical outcomes study: An application of methods for monitoring the results of medical care. *Journal of the American Medical Association, 262*, 925-930.

Chapter

5 Nursing Case Management

A Managed Care Organizational Strategy

Margaret M. Conger

[Case management means to] match the client with the most appropriate provider at the most appropriate time.

Mundt (1996)

The managed care era has brought with it the need for accountability for the use of limited health care resources. Nursing delivery systems have had to change to meet the economic and quality goals demanded by this increased accountability. An important change has been the development of the nurse case manager (NCM) role, which provides coordination of health services for clients in a time- and cost-effective manner. The focus of the NCM is to achieve well-defined client outcomes while using health care resources in an efficient manner. To accomplish these goals, the NCM must "match the client with the most appropriate provider at the most appropriate time" (Mundt, 1996, p. 50).

A number of experts (Lee, 1993; Weese, 1996) consider the nurse case manager (NCM) to be a pivotal person for meeting the cost-effective and quality goals of a managed care organization. These goals are met through strategies that lead to decreased organizational costs and improved health outcomes of clients served. One of these strategies that has been demonstrated to be effective in reaching these goals is the coordination of care services for clients who have been identified as at high risk for frequent need of hospitalization and other expensive medical services. These are often people with a chronic illness that, if not controlled, will result in the need for extensive medical expenditures. In this role, the NCM serves two clients—the patient requiring health care and the organization paying for and providing the care (Weese, 1996).

Coile (1995) has also identified the need to manage the care of a person with a chronic illness as vital to the success of a managed care organization. Without such management, scarce financial resources will not be controlled. He believes that the Advanced Practice Nurse (APN)—prepared as a clinician at the master of nursing level as a nurse practitioner or clinical nurse specialist—is the most appropriate person to manage this care. He also suggests that the APN is the most appropriate person to serve as the gatekeeper to make certain that patients are seen at the most appropriate care level.

Weese (1996), a physician who serves as a medical director of a managed care plan, sees the NCM as pivotal to the coordination of care of patients. He states, "Into this new universe that has the managed care environment as the key player, thankfully emerges the nurse case manager" (Weese, 1996, p. viii). He sees the NCM as serving the needs of several constituents. First, the NCM has an obligation to the employer, the managed care organization, to serve its needs as an employee of the organization. Secondly, the NCM has an ethical responsibility to the patient to ensure a high quality of care. And finally, the NCM must serve as a patient advocate, helping the client move through the organizational "red tape" that is so often part of a large organization. All of these authors see nursing case management as an opportunity for nursing to restructure its role, both within the acute-care hospital environment and within the larger community of subacute settings and community health settings.

Origins of Nursing Case Management

Some nurse experts see nursing case management as practiced within hospital settings as a new strategy (Gibb, Lonowski, Meyer, & Newlin, 1995; Zander, 1988). Others see it as a logical outgrowth of the primary nurse model described by Manthey (1991). However, nursing case management goes beyond the role originally envisioned for primary nurses. The expectation for delivery of care that is both cost and time efficient was not part of the primary care expectation. This value emerged with the movement into prospective payment under the Diagnosis Related Group legislation in the mid-1980s and is now imperative in the managed care environment.

Other differences also exist. In a primary nursing model, all patients admitted to the hospital are assigned a primary nurse. However, not all patients require nursing case management and thus will not be assigned a case manager. Criteria for selection for case management services will be discussed later in this chapter.

Another difference between primary nursing and case management is that the NCM moves beyond the traditional boundaries of a patient unit; the primary nurse remains within a unit framework. In most nurse case manager models, the patient is followed by the same nurse from the time of hospital admission to discharge and often back into the community (Manthey, 1991). This aspect of continuity of care is an important component of all case management models (Kurtin, 1995; Mundt, 1996). Thus the scope of responsibility for the NCM is greater than that of the primary nurse.

Other nurses see the role of the nurse case manager as coming out of a public health model (Mahn & Spross, 1996). This is particularly true of nursing case management as practiced in community settings. The early public health nurses focused on a wide range of concerns such as nutrition, sanitation, and education, as well as direct nursing care. An early example of such practice is found in the work of Lillian Wald in the Henry Street Settlement House in New York. The Henry Street nurses promoted health by looking holistically at individuals and families living within the larger community. This work expanded into an array of services, including first-aid clinics scattered around the city and school nursing services (Kalisch & Kalisch, 1986). These programs can be seen as early examples of what is now found in community nursing centers (Ethridge & Johnson, 1996; Hay, 1993). The work of Lillian Wald expanded into the provision of nursing services for enrolled members of the Metropolitan Life Insurance Company, first in New York City and then to many of the large eastern cities (Kalisch & Kalisch, 1986). Such activities can be seen as the precursors to the use of nurse case managers by modern-day health insurance companies.

Another link to the past for NCMs is the private duty nurse who, in the early part of the century, went into the patient's home and managed every aspect of care. This included nutrition, care of the environment, activities of daily living, and therapeutic interventions. Thus, although the NCM role has a new name, it has its origin in several early nursing delivery systems. Some have even suggested that nursing is finally returning to its own place in the community after almost a century of primary focus in the institutional setting (Hay, 1993; Manthey, 1991).

Definitions of Nursing Case Management

There are considerable differences in definitions of nursing case management (Powell, 1996). Some have suggested that case management is "whatever the institution defines it as" (Daniels & Sands, 1996). However, a general description of case management has been developed by the Case Management Society of America (1995). It states:

> Case management is a collaborative process which assesses, plans, implements, coordinates, monitors, and evaluates options and services to meet an individual's health needs through communication and available resources to promote quality cost-effective outcomes. (p. 2)

This definition fits most nurse case management programs.

Zander (1988) defines case management as "a model and set of technologies for the strategic management of cost and quality outcomes by clinicians who give care throughout an entire episode of illness" (p. 28). This definition fits case management as practiced within an acute-care hospital, but it needs to be broadened for practice outside of the hospital. Other definitions fit the wider arena in which case management often occurs. Yee (1990) states, "case management is the process of getting the right service to the right client" (p. 31). The American Nurses Association (ANA) (1992) definition states that "nursing case management is a health care delivery process whose goals are to provide quality health care, decrease fragmentation, enhance the client's quality of life, and contain costs" (p. 6).

In looking at these various definitions, some common elements emerge that can help as nursing is defining this new role. Ensuring quality of care is inherent in all of these definitions. The efficient provision of services, thus controlling costs, is also an important element in management of care. Because both quality and cost effectiveness are vital to the managed care environment, it is easy to see why the role for the NCM is growing so rapidly.

Models of Nurse Case Management

As nurse case management practice expands, a variety of models have emerged. These can vary both in the location in which they function and in the delivery system they use. The site of case management can be either "within the walls," an institutional form of case management, or "beyond the walls," a community-based approach. However, the basis for case management in all of these models is similar. It arises out of the nursing process, using the steps of assessment, planning, coordination of care, implementation of care, and evaluation. An emphasis of all case management programs is on the continuity of care across health care settings so that the timeliness and effective use of health care resources are maximized.

Acute-Care Nurse Case Management Models

The rise of case management within acute-care hospital settings has been very rapid in response to fiscal constraints placed on health care delivery by managed care organizations. The earliest of the acute-care hospital models was that at the New England Medical Center, Boston, Massachusetts, and it has served as a model for the development of many other hospital systems (Zander, 1988). Beyond-the-walls case management is an area of practice that is rapidly expanding, with a variety of community-based organizations that use nurse case managers constantly growing.

Within the hospital models there are a variety of structures. In many, such as at the New England Medical Center, the NCMs are unit based and provide direct patient care as well carrying a case load of patients for management only (Zander, 1990). These NCMs follow patients with a variety of medical conditions and move across units within the hospital and outpatient clinics as necessary. On some nursing units, the case manager oversees the care of patients with a variety of medical conditions. On other units, the patient population is quite specific, such as patients undergoing orthopedic procedures or cardiac surgery. Other acute-care nurse case management programs are population based, using criteria such as medical diagnosis or age group. For example, an NCM may follow only patients with similar medical conditions, such as those requiring cardiothoracic surgery or having respiratory disease. Other NCMs may see only babies and their families in a high-risk neonatal setting. The model as originally developed at the Tucson Medical

Center used both population-based case management and unit-based case management (Del Togno-Armanasco, Hopkins, & Harter, 1995).

The amount of direct "hands-on care" provided by the NCM differs among the various models. In most case management programs, the NCM is not the direct caregiver. In the model used at Hermann Hospital in Houston (Cohen & Cesta, 1993), direct patient care is given by staff, and the NCM coordinates and evaluates the care delivered. The delivery pattern at Sioux Valley Hospital (Koerner, Bunkers, Nelson, & Santema, 1989) also uses staff nurses as the primary caregivers; the NCM coordinates care for patients with complex health problems. However, in some programs, such as that used at the New England Medical Center (Zander, 1990), the NCM is the primary caregiver for the patient.

In a study of nurse satisfaction in an institution that modeled its case management program after the Zander model (Lynn & Kelley, 1997), significant dissatisfaction was found to be associated with the case management role related to the heavy staff nurse responsibilities. The case managers identified 75% of their time as spent on hands-on nursing activities and only 25% of their time as spent on case management activities. These nurses found it difficult to fully implement their new role because of the heavy direct patient care responsibilities included in the role. The staff nurses also found that their workload increased when they had to take over the management of patients assigned to the NCM when he or she left the unit to carry out case management functions. Thus, one must question the wisdom of including direct patient care responsibilities in the NCM role.

Community-Based Nurse Case Management Models

Nurse case management programs are rapidly spreading into community-based settings. Many of these programs have arisen out of acute-care-based programs. For example, the model developed at Carondelet St. Mary's in Tucson, Arizona incorporates both inpatient and community services. This model began with patients in acute-care settings and evolved into practice that occurs outside the hospital as well (Ethridge, 1991; Mahn, 1993). An innovative addition to this model has been the formation of a nursing HMO in which Medicare clients are followed by NCMs who coordinate services such as home health, intravenous therapy, homemaker, and respite care (Ethridge & Johnson, 1996). This model also uses community centers as points of service where NCMs can provide care to clients who are able to move about the community. For those clients who are homebound, the NCM will either make home visits or provide client and family support through telephone contact.

Another location for nurse case management is health insurance companies. The model used in these locations is that of a coordinator of care rather than direct hands-on care. The NCMs are expected to identify client needs, match these needs to the most appropriate resources, and then monitor the effectiveness of the services (Conti, 1996). The case management activities in these agencies are similar to other case management programs, but the way in which these activities are carried out differs. The coordination role is primarily one of referral to health care providers, both those within the agency and those contracted with the agency. The education role focuses a great deal on informing program members about their available benefits. Some clinical education is also included. The monitoring function is primarily that of making sure resources are used appropriately. Finally, the assessment function is that of determining what health care services a program member requires. Conti (1996) found in her study of these case managers located in health insurance companies that almost half of them were prepared at the associate degree level rather than baccalaureate or higher. This is in contrast with recommendations such as the ANA's (1992), in which the recommended preparation for this role is at least at the baccalaureate level.

Other community sites for nurse case management programs include government agencies, such as those found with the Medicaid program or with programs providing services to children with disabilities. Some NCMs work in community-based clinics that specialize in the care of a specific population such as a teen clinic or an HIV/AIDS outreach program. A growing number of nurses are developing nurse-managed businesses in which clients receiving workman's compensation benefits can be case managed. These specialized community sites for nurse case management will be explored in greater depth later in this book.

Goals of Nurse Case Management

The goals of nurse case management programs are similar despite individual programs' geographical location or physical setting. These goals are summarized in Table 5.1. A common major goal is early assessment of each client to ensure that services are provided in a timely and cost-effective manner.

TABLE 5.1 Goals of Nurse Case Management Programs

Early assessment results in
Timely provision of services
Services provided in low-cost setting
Early assessment of changes in client conditions
Empower clients to achieve
Optimal wellness
Self-directed care
Self-advocacy
Ability to make own decisions
Employee responses: Increase in
Productivity
Satisfaction
Retention

Another goal is the need for acute care to be reduced because of early assessment of changes in clients' conditions so that service can be provided in a lower cost setting (Powell, 1996). Finally, a goal to empower clients to achieve optimal levels of wellness and functioning is stressed (Powell, 1996). Closely associated with this is the goal of assisting clients to appropriately self-direct care, self-advocate, and make their own decisions to the greatest degree possible (Kurtin, 1995). Newell (1996) also suggests that an important goal of a case management program is to enhance employee productivity, satisfaction, and retention.

Mundt (1996) suggests that the entire case management process be focused on outcomes that are predetermined and constantly monitored. All care provided to clients must be resource efficient to achieve the needed financial goals of the provider agencies. At all times, the client must be connected with the "most appropriate provider at the most appropriate time" (p. 50).

A question often raised is whether nursing case management programs can achieve the fiscal goals that have been ascribed to them. Studies done at Carondelet St. Mary's in Tucson using a community-based nursing case management program to manage members of a Medicare Seniors plan provide some answers to this question. Data generated from this program indicate that the number of admissions, the length of stay, and the number of bed days for this population compared very favorably with data from other Medicare programs. For example, the average number of hospital bed days used by the population in the Carondelet system was 1,311, as compared to a Medicare national average of 2,798. Figuring that each bed day costs about $900.00 (1990 dollars), it can be seen that the use of nurse case management achieved significant savings (Ethridge, 1991).

A case management program developed within the Carondelet system for patients entering the hospital for elective coronary artery bypass grafting (CABG) also demonstrated significant savings (Mahn, 1993). In this program, the NCM coordinates the admission process and then follows the patient through the hospital stay. Postdischarge follow-up is done through telephone contact. Outcome analysis shows that the length of stay was reduced from 9 to 6 days in the case-managed group. An even more significant finding was that the number of readmission days within a 90-day period following discharge was only 3 days in the case-managed group, as compared to 30 days in the non-case-managed group. Again, the significance of these savings of health care costs is staggering.

Skills Required for Nurse Case Management

A number of skills required for a nurse to be successful in the role of the NCM are summarized in Table 5.2. An underlying skill needed is a strong clinical background in a particular segment of patient management so that the NCM is able to make appropriate clinical decisions. The nurse case manager must also be adept at the use of the nursing process. Very well-developed assessment skills are required, including the ability to do an in-depth biopsychosocial assessment. The ability to develop a plan of care that is individualized for each person is important. The implementation phase of the nursing process is more dependent on the ability of the NCM to work with others to accomplish the required care rather than the ability to provide direct care (Powell, 1996). The evaluation part of the nursing process is critical. With outcome assessment such a vital part of the managed care environment, case managers must learn to use evaluation tools effectively.

The NCM must be able to coordinate and manage care of clients across a continuum of care settings, interacting with a wide variety of health care providers. To do this, managerial competencies and organizational skills are necessary. The NCM must be able to identify and then communicate patient care needs clearly so that desired outcomes can be achieved. The ability of

TABLE 5.2 Skills Required for Nurse Case Management

Clinical skills in a specific area
Nursing Process
Assessment—biopsychosocial
Development of plan of care
Implementation of plan—able to work through others
Evaluation
Personal skills
Coordination abilities
Managerial and organizational abilities
Communication skills
Negotiation skills
Initiative
Autonomy
Vision for the future
Financial skills
Understand and use data
Understand sociological and political issues

the NCM to persuade others that the plan of care for a client is important to both the client and the larger organization is vital to achieving desired outcomes (Mundt, 1996). Both excellent communication skills and negotiation skills are also important to the NCM's success. The ability to function in an autonomous practice is also necessary to the success of the NCM. He or she must be able to take initiative in developing and executing a plan of care for a client. Many times the NCM will be developing new patterns of care and must be a self-starter. The NCM must also be able to envision a future for practice and not be afraid to alter the status quo if needed.

The frequency of each of these activities varies based on the location of the case manager. For example, in an acute-care agency, the case manager must be very competent in each of these areas. In an insurance company, the case manager tends to spend more time on the evaluation process. Also, the level of clinical knowledge will vary from one location to another. An NCM working with a cardiac surgery population must be very knowledgeable in managing this specific population. An NCM working in a community clinic must be familiar with a wide range of clinical problems to manage a variety of chronic diseases. Thus the setting of the case management will determine the specific needs of the case manager.

Skills that have historically been outside the domain of nursing are also required. These include a strong basis in fiscal health care management, the ability to understand and use financial data, and an understanding of both the sociological and the political issues inherent in health care management (Roberts-DeGennaro, 1993).

Who Is the Case Manager?

The term case manager has been used by a variety of providers in the health arena and has led to considerable confusion. Vocational counselors, social workers, life planners, and now nurses have all been in involved in case management. In acute-care health organizations, however, the traditional case managers have been social workers with a primary function of discharge planning (Powell, 1996). Nurses are increasingly used as case managers because of the pressures to move patients through the acute-care hospital more rapidly. The nurse is able to perform a clinical assessment and then use the data collected to begin the discharge plan at the time the patient is admitted. The dual ability to be both the assessor and the planner has made the nurse's skills invaluable in the case management role. Thus, the role of the discharge planner is being subsumed under nurse case management.

The answer to who should be the case manager cannot be categorically stated. Powell (1996) suggests that one must first examine the population to be served, identify the predominant needs of the population, and select the case manager who is knowledgeable about meeting these needs. In many organizations, the answer to this question has been to develop a combined social worker-nurse case management team in which each discipline takes responsibility for its respective areas of expertise (McNamara & Sullivan, 1995). With good communication between the team members, there is no need for the "turf wars" that have occurred in the past. Combining the strengths of the nurse with an excellent clinical knowledge and those of the social worker with an excellent understanding of community services can produce a winning situation for everyone (Powell, 1996).

Within the ranks of nursing, there are also differences. In the acute-care hospital, several different providers have been responsible for elements of care coordination. For example, the utilization review nurse (URN) has been a part of the acute-care setting for a number of years. This position developed out of the Peer Review Organization process mandated by the federal government to oversee both the cost-effectiveness and quality of care provided to

Medicare recipients. The role quickly spread to other payer groups such as health care insurance companies and, now, managed care organizations.

In the Medicare system, the URN was accountable for reviewing all Medicare admissions to make sure that the patient met appropriate diagnostic criteria for acute-care hospitalization. The URN was also responsible for assessing the need for continued hospitalization throughout the patient's hospital stay. This was often determined by the number and frequency of laboratory tests, intravenous medications, and other invasive treatments. The URN was also accountable for the condition in which the patient was discharged. If the discharge was premature and the patient was rehospitalized rapidly, the new event would be considered part of the initial hospitalization under the DRG system and no additional money would be provided for this care.

Faced with these responsibilities, the URN developed criteria for identifying at-risk patients who would either overstay the number of days available for reimbursement or require costly procedures. Often the criteria used by the URN were similar to those used by an NCM to identify patients requiring case management. Both providers followed the same patient, resulting in duplication of services. With the increase in fiscal restraints in health care, such duplication of services is not acceptable. Consequently, many hospitals are combining these roles into one to prevent such duplication (Daniels & Sands, 1996; Johnson & Proffitt, 1995). Nurses who have long worked in the utilization review role in which the major tool for obtaining information was the patient's chart are now retooling to develop the communication skills required to work directly with patients and families. NCMs, on the other hand, who come from a strong clinical background, must learn about insurance verification and all of the complexities of what constitutes an appropriate admission.

Educational Preparation for Nurse Case Management

The educational preparation needed for nurse case management has caused considerable debate. The level of education required by the agency for the nurse to perform nurse case management functions varies. Some agencies use nurses prepared at the associate degree level (Conti, 1996). Many require the nurse to be prepared at the baccalaureate level (Ethridge & Lamb, 1989; Zander, 1990). Others will only hire nurses with preparation at the master's level (Koerner et al., 1989).

Fralic (1992) points out that NCMs function in an unstructured environment and must be able to be comfortable in an arena of ambiguity, uncertainty, and change. Because of the autonomy required to carry out this role successfully, Mahn and Spross (1996) suggest that education at the advanced practice level achieved through obtaining a master's degree in nursing is needed to develop these abilities. Many other nurses agree with this recommendation (Connors, 1993; Hamric, 1992). In the differentiated practice, a model at Sioux Valley Hospital (Koerner et al., 1989), all nurse case managers are prepared at the graduate level. Trinidad (1993) suggests that the clinical nurse specialist (CNS) with a strong background in the care of patients within a particular diagnostic pattern is ideally suited for this role. The CNS has advanced clinical knowledge and skills to make appropriate assessments and determine patient-specific appropriate outcomes. The CNS also has experience in the leadership role required for effective coordination of services. The five identified roles of the CNS of expert practitioner, educator, researcher, administrator, and consultant are an excellent foundation for the NCM role.

The American Association of Colleges of Nursing (AACN) (1995) has developed criteria for education for APNs that can serve as a basis for planning a curriculum for nurse case managers. Their suggested graduate core curriculum includes courses in nursing theory, foundations of nursing practice, research, ethics, human diversity, and social issues. The suggested core curriculum also includes content on health care policy, organizational function, financing of health care, and professional role development. The guidelines also suggest that courses in health and physical assessment, pathophysiology, and pharmacology be included. With the strong foundation that such a curriculum can provide, the master's-prepared nurse should be well equipped to carry out the role responsibilities of the NCM.

The course work in the organization and financing of health care is an important part of this curriculum for the NCM. With the increased emphasis on accountability for both cost and quality outcomes, knowledge of insurance systems and financial strategies of the various managed care arrangements and the ability to evaluate options from a financial basis are important. Specific attention must also be paid to ensuring that the new graduate has a solid foundation in quality management techniques (Powell, 1996). Conger

(1996) suggests that education to assist graduates to work in a capitated environment, as opposed to a fee-for-service environment, is necessary. To make this shift, the nurse must undergo a role transformation.

The AACN (1996) also recommends that APNs become certified to demonstrate competency in the appropriate area of advanced practice. Such certification can be used to assure the public of the competency of the practitioner. Minimum qualifications for such certification are the completion of a master's degree in nursing, using the core curriculum components described above, and establishment of clinical competence in the appropriate area of practice.

In the area of nursing case management, such certification has been problematic. Up until October 1997, the only certification in case management was that offered by the Case Management Society of America. Because this certification was open to a variety of health care providers and could be obtained without the need for a master's degree in nursing, it does not meet the criteria listed above for advanced practice nursing. In 1997, the American Nurses Credentialing Center (Smith, 1997) introduced a case management exam that could be taken by nurses already holding certification in a core speciality. Thus, a nurse with master's preparation in a field such as medical-surgical nursing, gerontological nursing, or any of the clinical nurse specialist areas could add on certification in case management. This new opportunity for nurse case managers is a welcome addition to the legitimization of case management as a speciality field for nursing.

With the rapidity of growth in the case management field, it may not be practical to hold the educational standard of a master's degree in nursing as an entry level. Ethridge and Lamb (1989) conclude that a minimum of a baccalaureate education is needed to carry out nurse case manager competencies. Tucson Medical Center (Del Togno-Armanasco et al., 1995) also requires that case managers be prepared, at the minimum, at the baccalaureate level. Zander (1990), at the New England Medical Center in Boston, suggests that the BSN should be the minimum level of education for nurse case managers unless an individual demonstrates highly developed skills in nursing process, management, communication, and decision making. Finally, the ANA (1992) position statement on nurse case management recommends a baccalaureate degree in nursing as the minimum preparation for this position.

Perhaps one answer to this dilemma of educational preparation for nursing case management is to use baccalaureate-prepared nurses with expert clinical experience to function under the direction of an advanced practice case manager prepared at the master's level. In this way, the APN can serve as a role model and a mentor for the lesser prepared NCM. Another solution to the need for more master's-prepared nurses as case managers is to increase the educational opportunities for nurses. An increasing number of university programs are offering this as an area of concentration. Some of the very well-known programs in nurse case management are at the University of Arizona in Tucson and Villanova University in suburban Philadelphia.

Which Clients Require Case Management?

Criteria for determining who needs nurse case management is important in determining how best to use a scarce resource, the NCM. A number of nurses have developed criteria to be used as a preliminary screen for determining which clients require case management. An example of the types of conditions that suggest the need for case managment is shown in Table 5.3. Some common elements of these various screens include persons with chronic and/or destabilizing illnesses such as cardiac problems including hypertension, Chronic Obstructive Pulmonary Disease, diabetes, or cancer. People with these problems are in particular need of case management if their ability to manage the disease is impaired. A pattern of multiple hospital, emergency department, or clinic visits in a short time period is also a good indicator. Other factors that suggest the need for case management are problems with denial, depression, or anxiety about the health situation. Finally, problems associated with at-risk caregivers or lack of a caregiver are indicators that case management is needed. The client who has little or no social support has been shown to use health care services more than others. In two studies, single older women were found to have the longest hospital stays. This was attributed, in part, to the lack of family members to serve as caregivers (Lave & Leinhardt, 1976; Marchette & Holloman, 1986).

Screens for determining the need for case management services in community settings are also needed. Identification of high-risk members of a managed care organization is critical to control health care costs. This is particularly true because an HMO may get a large new group of enrollees at one time as a contract is finalized with a new company. A method is needed to rapidly assess the health needs of these new enrollees and identify those with health problems who require monitoring and management by an NCM.

TABLE 5.3 Screens for Case Management Services

Chronic and destabilizing disease
Cardiac
Respiratory
Diabetes
Cancer
Pattern of multiple
Hospital admissions
Emergency department visits
Clinic visits
Psychosocial problems
Denial
Depressions
Caregiver risk
Lack of caregiver

A system for evaluating health risk for enrollees in the managed care organization is under development at Carondelet St. Mary's nursing HMO (Lamb, 1995). Multiple levels of need are suggested. The lowest level is that of low risk for health needs. This group includes those who are able to provide self-care or have an existing support system in place. A person needs to be in stable health with or without chronic illness to be included in this category. This population will require only infrequent maintenance by the health organization. Enrollees who have required the services of case management in the past but now are in an improved health status may also be in this category. These enrollees can be managed very well through occasional educational programs and routine monitoring at infrequent times.

Enrollees in the moderate-risk category are those with a stabilized chronic disease who need no more than weekly maintenance in a community center. The nurse case manager functions as a "coach" to aid this population in appropriate health practices. The cost of this type of care is very minimal. The services of a community wellness center, a place to maintain health, are sufficient to meet the health needs of that population.

The next category for placement of enrollees is in the moderate- to high-risk group. These enrollees require direct contact with an NCM to assist them to learn to live with the chronic disease that has destabilized. For service at this level, the person cannot require more than weekly home visits. If the services of a NCM can be provided, this person can be maintained in the home setting. Without the services of an NCM, some type of institutional care may be required that will markedly increase the cost to the managed care organization.

The next level of need is that of requiring the services of Home Health Nursing. Criteria for care at this level of service includes a recent acute illness or an acute exacerbation of chronic disease. The need for visits is more than one per week and the person must be homebound. In addition, special technical skills provided by a nurse are needed. This level of care will be more costly to the managed care organization than that provided by the NCM. This population may need transitional care services in which around-the-clock nursing support is provided. Such care is best provided in an institutional setting.

The most cost-intensive service required in a community setting is that of hospice care. This is designed for those living with a terminal illness and who have an expected time frame for care that is short—less than 6 months. These enrollees require frequent assistance with care needs. They will need intense coordination of services by an NCM to manage the variety of health care workers who will be involved in their care.

Screening tools that can be used to rapidly identify the potential health needs of a newly enrolled population in a managed health care organization can serve a number of important functions. Cost and quality organizational outcomes can only be met when effective health monitoring programs are provided to those members at risk for development of acute or chronic health problems. One of the challenges of nurse case management programs is to develop screens for use in large managed care organizations to identify at-risk clients who would benefit from nurse case management services.

Conclusions

The practice of nurse case management is becoming pivotal to assuring the quality and cost-effective goals of managed care organizations. Thus it should not be surprising that it is a rapidly growing field for nurse practice in which nurses have the opportunity to reach a new level of professional competency. This is an exciting time in nursing—one in which nurses can reach out to new areas of practice and demonstrate their importance in the health care arena. The competencies needed to be successful in this field are great but within reach of the motivated nurse. This is the time to grasp the opportunity presented and grow into this new arena.

References

American Association of Colleges of Nursing. (1995). *The essentials of master's education for advanced practice nursing*. Washington, DC: Author.

American Association of Colleges of Nursing. (1996). *Position statement: Certification and regulation of advanced practice nurses*. Washington, DC: Author.

American Nurses Association. (1992). *Case management by nurses*. Washington, DC: Author.

Case Management Society of America. (1995). *Standards of practice for case management*. Little Rock, AR: Author.

Cohen, E. L., & Cesta, T. G. (1993). *Nursing case management: From concept to evaluation*. St. Louis, MO: Mosby.

Coile, R. C. (1995). Advanced practice nurse: A critical resource for managed care. *Health Trends, 7*(7), 1-7.

Conger, M. (1996). Integration of the clinical nurse specialist into the nurse case manager role. *Nursing Case Management, 1*(5), 230-234.

Connors, H. (1993). Impact of care management modalities on curricula. In K. Kelly & M. Mass (Eds.), *Managing nursing care: Promise and pitfalls* (pp. 190-207). St. Louis, MO: Mosby.

Conti, R. M. (1996). Nurse case manager roles: Implications for practice and education. *Nursing Administration Quarterly, 21*(1), 67-80.

Daniels, S., & Sands, J. (1996). Case management: A formula for resource conservation. *Journal of Healthcare Quality, 18*(1), 9-13.

Del Togno-Armanasco, V., Hopkins, L. A., & Harter, S. (1995). How case management really works. *American Journal of Nursing, 95*(5), 24I-24L.

Ethridge, P. (1991). A nursing HMO: Carondelet St. Mary's experience. *Nursing Management, 22*(7), 22-27.

Ethridge, P., & Johnson, S. (1996). The influence of reimbursement on nurse case management practice: Carondelet's experience. In E. L. Cohen (Ed.), *Nurse case management in the 21st century* (pp. 245-255). St. Louis, MO: Mosby.

Ethridge, P., & Lamb, G. (1989). Professional nursing case management improves quality, access, and cost. *Nursing Management, 20*(3), 30-35.

Fralic, M. (1992). The nurse case manager: Focus, selection, preparation, and measurement. *Journal of Nursing Administration, 22*(11), 13-14, 46.

Gibb, B., Lonowski, L., Meyer, P. J., & Newlin, P. J. (1995). The role of the clinical nurse specialist and the nurse manager in case management. *Journal of Nursing Administration, 25*(5), 28-34.

Hamric, A. B. (1992). Creating our future: Challenges and opportunities for the clinical nurse specialist. *Oncology Nursing Forum, 19*(Suppl. 1), 11-15.

Hay, M. (1993, October). Nursing's renaissance. *Health Progress, 74*(3), 26-32.

Johnson, K., & Proffitt, N. M. (1995). A decentralized model for case management. *Nursing Economics, 13*(3), 142-165.

Kalisch, P. A., & Kalisch, B. J. (1986). *The advance of American nursing*. Boston: Little, Brown.

Koerner, J. G., Bunkers, L. B., Nelson, B., & Santema, K. (1989). Implementing differentiated practice: The Sioux Valley Hospital experience. *Journal of Nursing Administration, 19*(20), 13-20.

Kurtin, S. E. (1995). Clinical tools for success in managing care. *Seminars for Nurse Managers, 3*(2), 100-107.

Lave, J., & Leinhardt, S. (1996). The cost and length of a hospital stay. *Inquiry, 13,* 327-343.

Lamb, G. S. (1995). Early lessons from a capitated community-based model. *Nursing Administration Quarterly, 19*(3), 18-26.

Lee, J. L. (1993). A history of care modalities in nursing. In K. Kelly (Ed.), *Managing nursing care* (pp. 20-38). St. Louis, MO: Mosby.

Lynn, M. R., & Kelley, B. (1997). Effects of case management on the nursing context: Perceived quality of care, work satisfaction, and control over practice. *Image: The Journal of Nursing Scholarship, 29*(3), 237-241.

Mahn, V. (1993). Clinical nurse case management: A service line approach. *Nursing Management, 24*(9), 48-50.

Mahn, V. A., & Spross, J. A. (1996). Nurse case management as an advanced practice role. In A. B. Hamric, J. A. Spross, & C. M. Hanson (Eds.), *Advanced nursing practice: An integrative approach* (pp. 445-465). Philadelphia: Saunders.

Manthey, M. (1991). Delivery systems and practice models: A dynamic balance. *Nursing Management, 22*(1), 28-30.

Marchette, L., & Holloman, F. (1986). Length of stay variables. *Journal of Nursing Administration, 165*(3), 12-19.

McNamara, S. T., & Sullivan, M. K. (1995). Patient care coordinators: Successfully merging utilization management and discharge planning. *Journal of Nursing Administration, 25*(11), 33-38.

Mundt, M. H. (1996). Key elements of nurse case management in curricula. In E. L. Cohen (Ed.), *Nurse case management in the 21st century* (pp. 48-54). St. Louis, MO: Mosby.

Newell, M. (1996). *Using nursing case management to improve health outcomes*. Gaithersburg, MD: Aspen.

Powell, S. K. (1996). *Nursing case management: A practical guide to success in managed care*. Philadelphia: Lippincott-Raven.

Roberts-DeGennaro, M. (1993). Generalist model of case management practice. *Journal of Case Management, 2*(3), 106-111.

Smith, M. (1997). ANCC to offer modular certification in nursing case management. *Credentialing News*. Retrieved September 4, 1998, from the World Wide Web: www.nursingworld.org/ancc/crednews.htm

Trinidad, E. (1993). Case management: A model of CNS practice. *Clinical Nurse Specialist, 7*(4), 221-223.

Weese, W. C. (1996). Forward. In S. K. Powell, *Nursing case management: A practical guide to success in managed care* (pp. viii-ix). Philadelphia: Lippincott-Raven.

Yee, D. L. (1990, July). Developing a quality assurance program in case management service setting. *Caring Magazine*, 30-35.

Zander, K. (1988). Managed care with acute care setting: Design and implementation via nursing case management. *Healthcare Supervisor, 6*(2), 27-43.

Zander, K. (1990). Managed care and nursing case management. In G. G. Mayer, M. J. Madden, & E. Lawrenz (Eds.), *Patient care delivery models* (pp. 37-62). Gaithersburg, MD: Aspen.

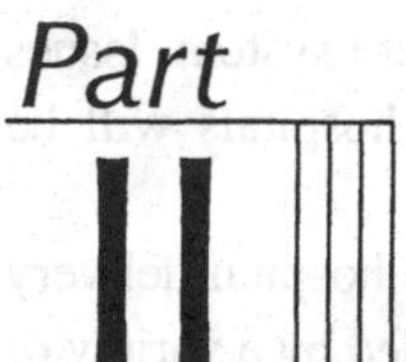

Part II Nursing Strategies in Acute-Care Hospitals

Desired outcomes of a managed care organization include the provision of health care that is both cost-effective and meets quality standards. Nurses are integral to achieving both of these goals. In this section of the book, strategies that nurses use in acute-care hospital settings will be explored.

Because nurses make up a large portion of the labor budget of any health care organization, both the role of the nurse and the number of nurses required to provide patient care have been areas for reevaluation. A variety of levels of health care workers have been introduced into the nursing staff, thus changing the skill mix. Issues related to this practice will be examined and strategies to improve health care delivery using the nurse extender will be discussed.

Another major change that has occurred in acute-care hospitals is the introduction of the nurse case manager. The complexities of managed care organizations have made it increasingly difficult for people to navigate the system to access needed services. Nurses have been found to be an excellent choice to assist people to navigate through the health care system. Issues related to the use of case management in acute-care hospitals will be explored.

A strategy that has become part of many acute-care hospital delivery systems has been the use of structured plans of care (called by a variety of titles). Perhaps the most common of these titles are *clinical pathway, critical pathway,* and *care map*. In this book, the title used will be *clinical pathway*. The use of a clinical pathway will be discussed, including its use as a tool for documentation of care provider interventions. Finally, strategies to measure resource utilization in the acute-care hospital will be explored.

Chapter

6 Use of Nurse Extenders

Margaret M. Conger

Nobody seemed to know where they came from, but there they were in the Forest: Kanga and Baby Roo. . . . "Here—we—are," said Rabbit very slowly and carefully, "all—of—us, and then suddenly, we wake up one morning and, what do we find? We find a Strange Animal among us. An animal of whom we have never even heard before!"

Winnie the Pooh (A. A. Milne)

Nurses are experiencing the discovery of a "strange animal" in their midst not too unlike what Pooh and his friends experienced. The nursing delivery system is undergoing profound changes, with the strange animal a new care provider, the unlicensed assistive person. The predominant nursing delivery system of the 1980s was that of either a primary care nursing system (Manthey, 1990) or total patient care in which the majority of care was provided by the registered nurse (RN). Many hospitals are now returning to a team approach more common in the 1960s and 1970s, with the use of nursing assistants and other unlicensed care providers to augment the RN staff. This change has caused tremendous concern among nurses. Apprehension about who is responsible for supervising this worker is widespread (Manuel & Alster, 1994; McKenna, 1995; Pedersen, Hoover, & Kisiel, 1995). Rather than approaching this change in health care delivery in fear as did Pooh and his friends, it is time to explore how this new worker can be incorporated into the workforce. We can learn from the end of Pooh's story:

> So Kanga and Roo stayed in the Forest. And every Tuesday Roo spent the day with his great friend Rabbit, and every Tuesday Kanga spent the day with her great friend Pooh teaching him to jump, and every Tuesday Piglet spent the day with his great friend Christopher Robin. So they were all happy again. (Milne, 1993)

With increased pressure placed on nursing managers to justify the need for an all RN staff that is considerably more expensive than a staff composed of a mix of various levels of care providers, hospitals are struggling to determine what skill mix is most effective in meeting both cost and quality outcomes. Many acute-care hospitals have brought in health care workers, called nurse extenders, who are trained at a lower level than the RN and paid a lower wage to meet cost goals. It is assumed that these new workers will be supervised by RN staff. Yet, little attention has been paid to how the RN staff will be prepared for this responsibility. In this chapter, the issue of who these new workers are and how they can best be used in health care delivery will be explored. Both professional and legal issues will be examined to help the RN develop an understanding of the responsibility entailed in supervising a nurse extender.

Reasons for Use of Nurse Extenders

The introduction of lesser trained health care workers as nurse extenders began in the late 1980s. Now, there are virtually no hospitals that do not use some type of RN substitution. In one study, 97% of the hospitals who reported data indicated that they had introduced some type of nurse extender into their nursing delivery system (Bostrom & Zimmerman, 1993). The reasons for this increased use of lesser skilled workers are several. In the late 1980s, a number of hospitals were reporting a nursing shortage (Eriksen et al., 1992; Neidlinger, Bostrom, Stricker, Hild, & Zhang, 1993). To manage this situation, administrators began to bring back a variety of health care workers to fill in for the RNs they were unable to hire.

As the movement to managed care increased in the 1990s, the reasons for bringing in alternate nursing staff changed. Concerns were raised about the amount of time RNs spent in "nonnursing" activities. In a study by Hayes

(1994), the types of nonnursing activities and the time spent in such activities were identified. Activities that were determined to be nonnursing included clerical or receptionist duties, errands off the unit, housekeeping tasks such as making beds, and dietary functions. This study also found a negative correlation between the amount of time spent in such nonnursing activities and job satisfaction of RNs. Other studies support that a significant amount of the RN's time is spent in nonessential care activities. Pedersen et al. (1995) found that the RNs spent 23% of their time on activities that did not require the skills of an RN. Grillo-Peck and Risner (1995) reported that 21.5% of the RN's time was spent on indirect care activities. Unfortunately, in these studies, different criteria were used to develop categories of nurse activity; thus it is difficult to compare the percentages between these studies. However, the pattern that emerges is that a significant amount of RN time is spent in activities that could well be done by a less expensive employee.

A third reason given for the move toward reducing the RN percentage of the nursing staff is cost. This reason has become extremely important as the move towards a capitated payment environment has increased. McKenna (1995) suggests that in financially hard-pressed times, skill substitution is an attractive management option. Many managers believe that there can be considerable cost savings by reducing the number of RNs and increasing the use of nurse extenders (Bostrom & Zimmerman, 1993). Thus, a critical issue in the present health care environment is how and by whom nursing care will be delivered. Perhaps the better question is, What is professional nursing care? What aspects of patient care require the skill of the RN? The role of the RN in the new health care delivery system will be explored in this chapter.

Who Is the Nurse Extender?

The use of nurse extenders in this country is not new. At various times during crises in health care delivery systems, workers prepared at less than the RN level have been brought into the workforce. During World War II, when there was an acute shortage of RNs, the licensed practical nurse (LPN) role emerged. The title for this person varies between states, with the majority using the title of licensed practical nurse and several using the title of licensed vocational nurse (LVN). The LPN (LVN) was prepared to provide bedside care under the direction of the RN. Another common health care provider is the certified nursing assistant (CNA). Both LPN (LVN) and CNA practices are regulated through legislative action at the individual state level.

Regulation of LPN and CNA Practice

For licensure as an LPN (LVN) in most states, the candidate must document completion of a prescribed course of study in an accredited school of practical nursing. For example, in California, the law states that the candidate must

> have successfully completed the prescribed course of study in an accredited school of vocational nursing or have graduated from a school which, in the opinion of the board, maintains and gives a course which is equivalent to the minimum requirements for an accredited school of vocational nursing in this state. (California Business and Professions Code Section 2866)

The scope of practice for the LVN is also defined by individual state statutes. For example, both Arizona statutes (Arizona Board of Nursing, Article 4, 1995, R4-19-401) and Oregon statutes (Oregon Revised Statutes, 1995, Section 678.010) specify that the LVN can plan, give nursing care, evaluate the effects of the care, and document the care provided to patients. Both states stipulate that this care must be provided under the supervision of a professional nurse or a physician. The California statute is somewhat more limiting in its definition of the scope of practice of the LVN (California Business and Professions Code Section 2859). This statute states that the LVN can perform services that require technical or manual skills that are taught in an accredited vocational nursing school. It also stipulates that this care must be provided under the supervision of a licensed physician or a registered professional nurse. The scope of practice for the LPN (LVN) has expanded in recent years. Many states now allow the LPN (LVN) to administer oral and some parenteral medications. More recently, the management of intravenous therapy has been added to the role if the LPN takes additional training.

Legislative standards have also been established to define the practice role of CNAs. Oregon is quite specific in stating that "nursing assistants be adequately trained" (Oregon Revised Statutes, 1995, Section 678.440). The Oregon State Board of Nursing is charged with both developing a curriculum and standards for a training program for nursing assistants and for certifying examinations (Oregon Revised Statutes, 1995, Sections 678.440 and 678.442). Arizona is similar in its requirements for nursing assistants. In this state, the nursing assistant candidate must complete a program approved by the board and satisfactorily complete a competency exam (Arizona Board of Nursing, Article 4, 1995, R4-32-1645). The curriculum in a nursing assistant program that meets the Arizona State Board of Nursing requirements includes topics such as provision of basic hygiene, meeting nutritional needs, providing for a safe environment, positioning and transferring of patients, and measuring vital signs. It also includes management of simple procedures such as use of heat and cold, prevention and treatment of pressure ulcers, use of restraints, and care of patients with a Foley catheter (Coconino Community College, 1998).

Current Use of LPNs and CNAs

As part of the nursing shortage of the late 1980s and the cost reduction constraints arising in the 1990s, large numbers of LPNs and CNAs have been brought back into the acute-care hospital workforce to fill positions formerly held by RNs. However, they are now being used in new ways. In one hospital, LPNs were introduced into the intensive care unit to supplement the RN staff (Eriksen et al., 1992). The rationale given for this decision was that the LPN had both training and experience in patient care, and thus the expected orientation time would be less than if an untrained worker was used. There was a ready supply of LPNs available from the schools in the local area. All job candidates went through a nursing course in which the skills and assessments required to care for critically ill patients were taught both in classroom and clinical experiences. Stanford University Hospital (Bostrom & Zimmerman, 1993) also introduced LPNs into the workforce to assist the RN on the night shift. CNAs were used as the nurse extender during the other shifts.

Many other institutions are using CNAs as the nurse extender. However, their job descriptions are being revised to include an expanded list of tasks (Bostrom & Zimmerman, 1993; Hayes, 1994; Hines, 1994; Johnson, 1995; Pedersen et al., 1995). In all of these situations, the nursing assistant had some formal education and had demonstrated clinical experience as part of the hiring requirement as well as having passed a certification examination.

Because both the CNA and the LPN have well-established roles based on standardized educational programs and licensing or certification exams, there is a general understanding of their capabilities. However, a new level of worker has been recently introduced, the unlicensed assistive person (UAP). The role for this level of worker is varied based on each institution's job description. There are no established criteria for training programs or examinations to determine a minimal level of competency for the UAP; each hospital determines the desired educational level.

The job descriptions for UAPs who have direct patient care responsibility generally include basic care functions such as assistance with hygiene needs, nutrition, respiratory care, vital sign measurements, specimen collection, and basic documentation (Grillo-Peck & Risner, 1995). The area in which their responsibilities have increased is in the addition of some bedside testing techniques, such as electrocardiograph testing and blood draws for laboratory specimens. The responsibilities commonly ascribed to the nurse extender role are shown in Table 6.1.

Many institutions have hired CNAs for this position and then have provided additional training in certain tasks such as laboratory specimen collection and specialized testing (Pedersen et al., 1995). Other institutions have hired persons with no nursing experience at all and then provided minimal training within the institution (Grillo-Peck & Risner, 1995). For example, at a large medical center in California, UAPs with no previous nursing experience were hired to partner with the RNs (Neidlinger et al., 1993). The reason given for this decision was to prevent role preconceptions among the newly hired staff. These UAPs were provided with 2 days of classroom instruction and then 2 weeks of clinical orientation working with an RN while delivering care. Evaluation of the program found that the limited amount of classroom education placed a great burden on the RN staff, which had to do the clinical training. The recommendation for future programs was either to develop a longer classroom training period or hire CNAs who already had some experience with patient care activities.

Another group of workers in the UAP classification is that of patient service associate (PSA), as described by Kieltyka, Robertson, and Behner (1997) and Grillo-Peck and Risner (1995). The job description for this level of worker is a combination of housekeeping duties, assisting patients with nourishments, stocking supplies, transporting patients, and assisting the RN with simple care tasks. In interviews with some newly hired PSAs, Gordon (1997) found that institutional training programs were minimal. One worker reported that he had been a janitor in a skilled nursing facility, went to a 2-hour class on basic patient care procedures, and was then expected to participate

TABLE 6.1 Areas of Responsibility: Unlicensed Assistive Personnel

Hygiene needs
Nutrition
Respiratory care
Vital sign measurements
Specimen collection
Provision of a safe environment
Client positioning and transfer techniques
Prevention and treatment of pressure ulcers
Basic technical procedures
Use of heat and cold
Use of restraints
Foley catheter care
Simple dressing techniques
Simple bedside testing
ECG testing
Blood draws
Basic documentation of care

in activities such as patient transport. With each institution free to develop training standards, it is possible to have workers providing patient care with a questionable level of expertise.

Educational Programs for Unlicensed Nurse Personnel

With the introduction of the UAP in hospitals across the country, standards for developing educational programs for their training are needed. The program at Good Samaritan Hospital in Cincinnati, Ohio is an example of the content that should be included in such programs (Esselman, 1995). Basic nursing aid responsibilities such as bedmaking, hygiene measures, vital signs, height and weight, and mobility issues were taught. Also simple procedures such as uncomplicated dressing changes, enemas, specimen collection, running a 12-lead electrocardiograph machine, and gastrostomy tube feedings were also included. The course lasted for 6 weeks, with 4 weeks of classroom and clinical laboratory time and the last 2 weeks in direct patient care under the direction of the RN. In the first group of participants, only four of the twelve in the group had previous nurse aid experience. The others were drawn from other health-related fields.

In other institutions that require potential UAP candidates to have basic nurse aid certification prior to hire, the focus of the training program is on developing advanced technical skills. These include blood draws for clinical specimens, some respiratory techniques such as oxygen administration by nasal cannula, and using a 12-lead electrocardiographic machine. Many of these skills come from the domain of the medical assistant role. O'Brien and Stepura (1992) describe a 3-day course in which such skills were taught. They found that CNAs who were able to perform some of these advanced skills were more useful as RN partners than a CNA with only the skills normally taught in a CNA program.

The cost-effectiveness of each hospital developing and administering a training program for UAPs is an important consideration. Is it reasonable for each facility to develop its own course, or would it be more cost-effective to centralize the needed training in a different setting? The experience reported by Neidlinger et al. (1993) would suggest that hiring CNAs who had received training in recognized nursing assistant programs is more cost-effective than developing training programs within each hospital. Some community colleges are beginning to add content to their basic nurse assistant training to include some of the skills required of the UAP. Perhaps as this movement continues, a standardized educational program will be developed and some type of certification program will be required for this level of worker. Such a movement would certainly add credibility to the role.

What Is the Role of the RN When Working With the UAP?

In today's managed care environment, the traditional role of the RN of providing total patient care within the acute-care hospital is probably gone. Use of an all-RN staff is believed by many to be too expensive (Barter, McLaughlin, & Thomas, 1997; Hendricks & Baume, 1997; Neidlinger et al., 1993). Instead, a staff mix of RNs and a variety of lesser skilled care providers has become the accepted practice. New practice patterns for the RN are needed when working with the UAP as a partner in providing patient care. Before redesigning the work of nurses, careful consideration must be given to determining the ratio of RNs to nurse extenders. In all situations, the RN remains accountable for the standard of patient care (Joel, 1994). With these rapid shifts in the delivery of nursing care, it is important to evaluate what aspects of patient care must be retained by the RN and what can be delegated to the UAP. The top consideration must be the delivery of safe patient care along with meeting the cost constraints of the managed care organization. Unfortunately, this has not always been the case. Manuel and Sorensen (1995) report that a California hospital has proposed a plan to use only one RN to supervise nurse extenders on patient units of 24 to 30 patient beds. Similar patterns using large numbers of UAPs are emerging across the nation (Burtt, 1997). One must question whether when using such staffing patterns, patient safety can be maintained.

Professional Responsibilities

Coile (1995) suggests that, in the managed care environment, the RN will become a nurse case manager who will coordinate patient care and will delegate assignments to nonregistered nurses. The use of the term *nurse case manager* here is probably not the best term when one considers the wider definition of a nurse case manager. A better term used for this function is *care coordinator*. In Coile's view, the RN will lead teams of lesser skilled caregivers in which delegation activities are paramount. The RN responsibilities will be to assess patients, develop care plans, continuously monitor quality, manage costs and resources, and, at the same time, achieve high customer satisfaction.

Gordon (1997) has a very different view of the RN role. Professional nursing includes the ability to assess and respond appropriately to complex health situations. To do this, the RN must have excellent assessment skills, focus on the primary patient issues, and be able to make critical judgments. The RN must also be able to negotiate with other caregivers to provide an environment in which patient care needs can be met using multiple providers. These skills cannot be reduced to a list of nursing tasks. A similar analysis of RN responsibilities has been reported by Pedersen et al. (1995). Professional RN responsibilities include those activities that require critical thinking skills, such as assessment of client status and situation and crisis intervention. Activities mandated by legal and philosophical thought and continuing education activities were also identified as within the domain of professional nursing (Pedersen et al., 1995). These characteristics of professional responsibilities are shown in Table 6.2.

TABLE 6.2 Professional Registered Nurse Responsibilities

Assessment skills
Identify patient issues
Critical judgment making
Knowledge of appropriate actions
Communication skills
Negotiation skills
Crisis intervention
Critical thinking
All interventions legally mandated

Gordon (1997) gives several examples that demonstrate the need for the RN in the patient care situation. In one situation, a woman experienced an anaphylactic response to an intravenous drug administration that resulted in a respiratory arrest. The RN quickly called the "code" and provided oxygen and an antihistamine. The patient was breathing by the time the physician arrived in the unit. In another situation, a woman with end-stage cancer was in extreme pain and indicated to the RN that she was ready to die. Her family was not ready to accept her death and wanted all possible treatment done. The RN negotiated with patient, family, and physician to provide treatment to keep her pain level under control and let her die as she requested. The RN also negotiated with the physician to order a foley catheter to prevent discomfort when using a bedpan. These examples illustrate the need for an RN to be present with patients to provide quality nursing care. This is not the work of an unskilled person.

Similarities to Team Nursing

A question to consider is, What are the similarities between the present use of an RN–nurse extender dyad and the team-leading structure common in the 1960s and 1970s? Lyon (1993) sees the present movement in health care delivery as a return to the team nursing process. In the team-leading model, the RN assesses patients, plans care based on patient needs and priorities, supervises caregivers, allocates resources, and provides the care that lesser skilled assistive personnel are not capable of doing. Some nurses fear that a return to a team nursing delivery system will lead to the same problems experienced earlier when the focus of care was on tasks, not the patient (MacLeod & Sella, 1992; Townsend, 1994). These authors suggest that the team nursing method of the past resulted in care provided by multiple persons with no one person taking accountability for the outcome of the care. The composition of the team continually shifted, which prevented development of trust among the team members. The team method resulted in little continuity of care because each team member focused on a specific function. The end result was a patient who did not know what to expect from each of the several caregivers.

With the movement into the use of multiple levels of caregivers, new strategies are needed to prevent the problems common to the old team nursing delivery system. Accountability for patient care must remain the responsibility of the RN. The RN must also remain as the decision maker regarding patient care. The ratio of RN to nurse extenders must be in a range that permits the RN to be able to assess, plan, and evaluate the care of each patient managed by the team. One must question how this can happen if the RN is overseeing more than one or at the most two nurse extenders at a time.

Townsend (1994) suggests strategies to use to develop team members when adding the UAP to the care delivery system. These are based on building relationships among team members, expanding each team member's clinical expertise, and increasing trust among team members. Familiarity can be developed by having the RN partner participate in the selection and orientation process for the nurse extender. Also, maintaining consistency in working groups by having the nurse extender work with only one or two RNs rather than a different RN each shift will help establish familiarity. The expertise level of the nurse extender is developed through well-established training programs followed by demonstrated competency of skills. Trust can be enhanced by knowing the partner's competency and developing clear delineation of roles. Effective communication skills, including conflict management and negotiation skills, are also essential to the process.

Education Needed for Registered Nurses for Effective Teamwork

To successfully implement a nursing delivery system in which nurse extenders will be used to assist the RN, educational programs need to be offered to upgrade the knowledge and skill level of the RN in three areas. These are enhanced communication skills, delegation decision making, and process strategies for working in a partnership relationship.

Communication Skills

An important aspect of working in a partnership relationship with another worker is skill in communication. Pender (1992) discusses the need for negotiation skills when working in any type of partnership. Conflict management is another important skill when supervising others. The ability to negotiate effective compromises when working with others can lead to win-win solutions when conflict arises. Clarity in communication with these partners must also be learned.

Hospitals that have instituted care systems using nurse extenders report that the need for communication skills for nurses has increased. O'Brien & Stepura (1992) found that when working with nurse extenders, more explicit and concrete communication was needed than when working with an all-RN staff. In a study by Manuel and Sorensen (1995), nurse managers rated leadership and communication skills as very important for new nursing graduates entering the workforce. These were rated as highly as the need for more traditional skills, such as patient assessment and clinical technical competency, for these new RNs. The need for increased communication skills was attributed to the changing skill mix found in patient care delivery systems. Thus, when a hospital decides to bring in nurse extenders, serious consideration must be given to developing training programs in communications skills for the RN staff.

Delegation Decision Making

The increased use of nurse extenders in the workforce has sparked interest in how RNs can be taught the delegation skills so vital to providing quality of care for patients (Erlen, Mellors, & Koren, 1996). However, many health care institutions have not used a systematic process to teach this skill (Barter et al., 1997; Russo & Lancaster, 1995). Also, few nursing programs include delegation decision making for working with nursing assistive personnel in the educational experience of the students (Barter et al., 1997; Freidman, 1990; Manuel & Sorensen, 1995). To prepare both current and future nurses to function effectively when working with nurse extenders, new teaching strategies must be developed.

Delegation has been defined as the act of transferring responsibility for the performance of a task from one person to another (Arizona Nurses Association, 1992). It is presumed that the delegator has greater knowledge than does the person to whom the task is delegated. The delegatee is responsible for only a part of the greater whole; the delegator retains accountability for the entire process.

Delegation of nursing activities is a skill that most nurses did not learn in their basic nursing education program. Most student nurses use a total patient care process in their clinical experiences. Also, because various models of total patient care have been the major delivery system in the recent past, there are no role models available for the nurse to use to learn delegation skills on the job. Thus, it is not surprising that when hospitals plan a change to bring in nurse extenders, RNs have expressed the need for formal instruction in this area.

Delegation cannot be taught by learning a list of tasks that can be performed by the nurse extender. Rather, the focus of learning needs to be on how to assess the needs of each patient and, then, how to determine which of the nursing tasks required can be safely carried out by the assistant. In a study in a large university medical center, the ability of the RN to delegate to the nurse extender was found to be inconsistent (Russo & Lancaster, 1995). The less experienced RNs were more reluctant to give up some of the nonnursing tasks than were the more experienced nurses. Their recommendation was that when RN-UAP partnerships are formed, more experienced RNs should be chosen for the role. They did not see delegation to UAPs as an appropriate activity for the new RN. However, in most hospital situations, the inexperienced RN is expected to work with a UAP just as is the more experienced RN.

Nurses must be very vigilant in determining what lies within the RN's scope of practice. A number of legal and regulatory groups have developed guidelines for principles for delegation. The educational programs established for teaching delegation should include these principles. The National Council of State Boards of Nursing (1995) has developed a position paper on delegation principles. As part of their position paper, they have developed the following "Five Rights of Delegation":

1. The right task
2. The right circumstances

3. The right person
4. The right direction/communication
5. Right supervision (p. 4)

The National Council of State Boards of Nursing (1995) has identified as a primary concern in delegation decision making the "protection of the health, safety, and welfare of the public" (p. 1). Also, the accountability for this decision making remains with the RN. This position paper also supports the concept that nursing cannot be reduced to a list of tasks; rather, nursing comprises assessment, evaluation, and judgment that goes beyond the task level. Delegation criteria in this statement include the authority to delegate, as stated by the nurse practice act, and qualifications of both the delegator and the delegatee. The registered nurse must assess the situation, including the needs of the patient, the setting in which the situation occurs, and the available resources. Then the nature of the task to be delegated must be considered in terms of the skill, knowledge, and demonstrated competence of the delegatee. If the delegatee has all of these, the task can be delegated. However, the RN retains accountability to supervise performance of the task and to evaluate the outcome.

Educational programs aimed at teaching delegation to a nurse extender must include a component on the specific state regulatory statutes for nursing practice. These statutes will determine the areas of responsibility for all RNs. Most state statutes provide for the RN to legally delegate tasks to a lesser skilled person. For example, the Arizona Board of Nursing Statutes (1995) state that the scope of practice for the registered nurse includes "directing and evaluating of nursing care provided by other licensed nurses and other personnel" (p. 1). The practice of professional nursing in California is described as

> Giving direct nursing care to each patient according to needs or assigning these functions to assistants in accordance with the preparation and competency of the available staff. (California Code of Regulations, Section 1443)

The law for delegation by licensed practical nurses is less clear. Many states have statutes that define LPN practice in terms of specific tasks that are included in their educational programs. If delegation is not defined in the law, the LPN cannot legally delegate tasks to an assistant. The law is also quite clear in stating that the person to whom a task is delegated cannot in turn delegate the task to another person.

The Arizona Nurses Association (1992) has developed a position paper on the use of unlicensed assistive personnel to guide practice in this area. The following principles are recommended for use when delegating to a UAP. First, the RN remains accountable for all care provided to the client. The RN is accountable for the assessment of the patient's needs and conditions, development of the plan of care, and evaluation of outcomes from the care provided. Second, a task cannot be delegated to a UAP unless he or she both has the education for and has demonstrated competence in that task. If the delegated task is within the demonstrated competence of the UAP, he or she will be accountable for the outcome of the care provided, but the RN retains overall accountability for the patient.

Although the development of a list of tasks that can be performed by a UAP may seem to be a solution to delegation decision making, this may not be the most appropriate approach to take. Yet the pressure to do just that is strong. For example, nurses at Brigham & Women's Hospital in Boston, Massachusetts were asked by their administration to draw up a list of tasks that could be performed by UAPs. To prevent this from happening, they had to threaten to strike. The language finally used as the result of contract negotiation was that the RN had sole discretion in delegating tasks to the UAP. The delegation decision would not be based on a list of tasks but would be determined after an assessment of patient needs (Burtt, 1997).

The California Board of Registered Nursing (1994) has also developed a position paper on the use of nurse extenders that is quite specific in how the delegation process should be conducted. In addition to specifying an RN role that is similar to those already discussed in terms of assessment, planning, and evaluation of care, emphasis is placed on the patient's condition. This statement limits the care of medically fragile patients to the RN no matter what the task capabilities of the nurse extender might be. *Medically fragile* is defined as a "patient who is experiencing an acute phase of an illness, or is in an unstable state that would require an ongoing assessment by a registered nurse" (p. 5). This statement also addresses the need for a sufficient number of RNs to be present so that the direct-care RN is able to make decisions about each patient.

Principles for delegation decision making can be derived from these guidelines. A model that outlines these steps is shown in Figure 6.1. First, the task must be within the guidelines developed by the state board of nursing. For example, administration of medications by the intravenous route cannot be done by an unlicensed person. Secondly, the task must be within the job description for the nurse extender as developed by the institution. Finally, the task to be delegated must be within the educational preparation and demonstrated competency of the nurse extender. If the nursing function to be delegated falls within each of these parameters, the nurse can consider delegating it to the nurse extender. However, one must then consider the problems the patient is experiencing in the biological, psychosocial, and spiritual areas. The patient must be in a stable medical condition to have an unlicensed person provide care (stable has been defined as not medically fragile). If any of these areas are unstable, the RN must either retain those nursing functions related to the problem or provide the nurse extender with specific instructions about the management of the problem. When all of these considerations are evaluated, a delegation decision can safely be made.

An example of how these principles can be used is illustrated in the situation of Robert, a 72-year-old man who had just been admitted to the hospital with a cerebral vascular accident. A regular dinner tray had been ordered for Robert and was about to be brought to his room by a UAP. The RN stopped the UAP and told her that she needed to assess Robert's swallowing ability before he could eat. In this situation, providing for Robert's nutritional needs was within the scope of practice for the UAP; however, the patient's condition had first to be assessed by the RN. It turned out that Robert had a great deal of difficulty in swallowing and needed to be placed on a nothing-by-mouth order until his condition improved. Delegating nutritional care to the UAP prior to assessment of patient condition could have resulted in serious harm to Robert.

Process Strategies

The third area of education for RNs when developing partnership models of nursing is the process of managing workload. To develop effectively functioning teams, a methodology for how the workload assignment will be managed must be learned. Certain practices have been demonstrated to enhance team effectiveness. O'Brien and Stepura (1992) describe the process used in their institution. The RN and nurse extender work together as a dyad. The process starts with the RN receiving reports on the assigned group of

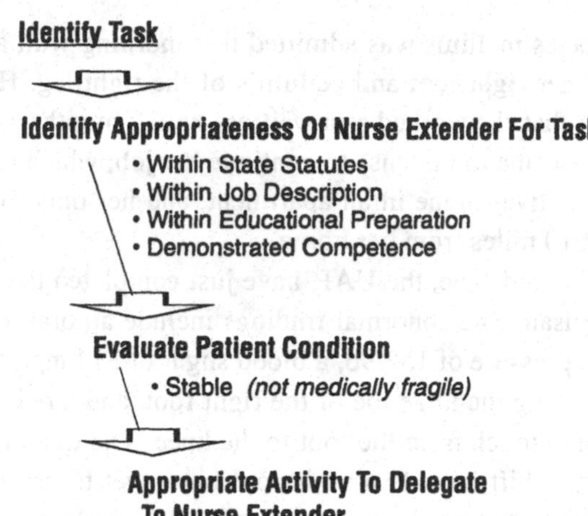

Figure 6.1 Model for Delegation Decision Making

patients. The RN and the assistant, the nurse technician (NT), then make rounds on all of the assigned patients and do a beginning-of-shift assessment. They then determine target goals for the shift and individual responsibilities. The communication between the dyad is continuous, so there are no surprises at the end of the shift. In this process, patient changes can be quickly assessed and dealt with. Because the RN and NT are a pair that always work together, a great deal of trust is developed. Each member of the dyad knows each other's work habits, capabilities, and routine.

Teaching the process of working in a partnership relationship is an important part of the educational program. To do this effectively, both classroom and clinical instruction time are needed (Hansten & Washburn, 1997; Manuel & Sorensen, 1995). As more nurses learn to carry out effective partnerships with RNs and nursing extenders working side by side, it is hoped that role models will develop and can serve as guides for new nurses in this new nursing delivery system.

Clinical Example

To illustrate the principles presented in this chapter, the following clinical example is provided. Susan, a 59-year-old woman with a 30-year history of adult onset diabetes mellitus was admitted this morning with an abscess on the large toe of her right foot and cellulitis of the right leg. Her admission history indicates that she worked as a waitress until 2 months ago, when pain in her right leg became too intense to continue her job, which required her to stand all day. She lives alone in an apartment, and her only family is a son who lives about 10 miles from her home.

Tom, the RN, and Jane, the UAP, have just completed the evening shift assessment of Susan. The abnormal findings include an oral temperature of 101.2 F, a blood pressure of 152/96, a blood sugar of 314 mg/dl, drainage on the dressing covering the large toe of the right foot, and a red, swollen right leg that is warm to touch from the foot to the knee. The treatment orders for Susan during this shift include a whirlpool bath, wet-to-dry normal saline dressings to the infected toe, bedrest except for the whirlpool treatment, and vancomycin 1000 mg in a 250 ml piggyback solution to be given after an IV is started. She is also to have 6 units of NPH insulin before her evening meal and a finger stick for blood glucose levels to determine the need for regular insulin to be given on a sliding scale regimen. She has a 1,600-calorie American Diabetic Association diet ordered that includes both her evening meal and a bedtime snack.

With this information, Tom begins to develop a plan for managing Susan's care. His first step is to discuss with Jane her knowledge about managing a whirlpool bath and dressings changes while maintaining appropriate infection control strategies. Jane assures him that she has done these procedures many times and feels competent to manage the treatments. However, Tom is concerned about evaluating the status of the abscess on Susan's toe and asks Jane to let him know when she has Susan in the whirlpool bath so that he can observe the site. He also asks Jane to report to him about the amount of the evening meal that Susan eats because of her apparent uncontrolled blood sugars and the need for her bedtime snack because of the NPH insulin she will be receiving.

Tom also plans with Jane about the timing of the treatments that will be done during the evening shift. He decides that starting an intravenous line is the first priority of the shift so that Susan can be started on her intravenous antibiotic as soon as possible. Tom will also need to do a finger stick for a blood glucose level around 5:00 p.m., prior to her dinner being served, to determine if regular insulin will be needed in addition to her NPH insulin.

The problems that Tom has identified as important to Susan's care are:

Tasks	Rating	Problems
Initial shift assessment	RN & NE	Impaired skin integrity R/T abscess on toe
Serve dinner and assess intake	NE with instruction	At risk for infection transmission R/T use of whirlpool bath
Bedtime snack	NE	Knowledge deficit R/T diabetic management
Whirlpool bath	NE with instruction	Impaired mobility R/T pain, infection right foot
Dressing changes	NE with instruction	Impaired self-care management R/T lack of support systems
Start IV	RN	
Administer IV antibiotic	RN	
Insulin administration	RN	
Blood glucose checks	RN	
Initiate discharge plan	RN	

Figure 6.2 Results of Delegation Decision Making
NOTE: NE = nurse extender; R/T = related to.

1. impaired skin integrity related to abscess on toe
2. knowledge deficit related to diabetic management
3. at risk for infection transmission related to use of common facilities (the whirlpool bath)
4. impaired mobility related to pain, infection of right foot
5. at risk for impaired self-care management related to lack of support systems

His assessment of Susan's ability to manage her situation is very low; also her knowledge about diabetes management appears to be very low. He is not sure about her motivation to take more responsibility for her self-care. Because of this assessment, Tom plans to find some time during his shift to talk with Susan to better develop a plan of care that will be directed to enhance Susan's self-care abilities.

Even though Susan has just been admitted to the hospital, Tom knows that plans for her discharge must be initiated immediately. He has concerns about her ability to return home to live independently because of a possible prolonged healing time for her wound. He wants to start discussion with Susan's son about possible alternatives for her care. To do this, he alerts Jane to let him know if Susan's son comes in to visit during the evening shift. Figure

6.2 illustrates Tom's decisions about what tasks related to Susan's care can be delegated to Jane, the nurse extender, and which he must retain. It also indicates the problems identified that affect his delegation decisions.

This clinical example also illustrates both the communication needed between the RN and the nurse extender and the organizational processes used to work effectively as a dyad. Tom does not assume that Jane can manage the wound care needed for Susan just because wound care is an expected competency of a nurse extender in this institution. He clarifies the importance of Jane's blood sugar check prior to the evening meal. He is also clear about needing to be told when Susan is in the whirlpool bath so he can check the status of her wound and needing to be told if Susan's son comes in to visit. With this clear communication, Tom has established an environment in which Susan will receive quality nursing care in a cost-effective manner.

Conclusions

The introduction of a variety of nurse extenders is an emerging part of the managed care environment. The reasons for this change are many, including both cost issues as well as the desire to have professional nurses devote their time to truly professional activities. With the influx of a variety of new health care workers into the acute-care hospital setting, the issue of delegation of nursing tasks has become an important consideration. A pressing need is the education of RNs so that effective delegation decisions can be made. Only by providing such education can the safety and welfare of the public be protected.

In reviewing the work that has been done on establishing principles for effective delegation decision making, a case can be made that the use of nurse extenders should not affect the quality of patient care as long as these principles are followed. Thus, with appropriate education and experience, the RN can learn to use the nurse extender in an effective manner. However, nurses will need to be educated and supported in this process. It takes considerable professional judgment to make this system work effectively. It remains the individual responsibility of each RN to understand the scope of practice of both self and nurse extender and to remain within legal boundaries of practice. Appropriate delegation decision making is vital to provide for the safe and effective care of each patient.

References

Arizona Board of Nursing. (1995). *Title 4. Professions and occupations (Chapter 19, Article 4. Regulation).* Retrieved August 4, 1998, from the World Wide Web: http://www.state.az.us/bn/html/rules.html

Arizona Nurses Association. (1992). *Position statement on the use of unlicensed assistive personnel when under the direction of the registered nurse.* Phoenix, AZ: Author.

Barter, M., McLaughlin, F., & Thomas, S. (1997). Registered nurse role changes and satisfaction with unlicensed assistive personnel. *Journal of Nursing Administration, 27*(1), 29-38.

Bostrom, J., & Zimmerman, J. (1993). Restructuring nursing for a competitive health care environment. *Nursing Economics, 11*(1), 35-41.

Burtt, K. (1997, March/April). Dangerous trends in health care galvanize nursing community. *American Nurse, 29*(2), 1, 6.

California Board of Registered Nursing. (1994). Board issues advisory statement on unlicensed assistive personnel. *BRN Report, 7*(2), 1, 3.

Coconino Community College. (1998). *Course syllabus: Nursing assistant I.* Flagstaff, AZ: CCC Nursing and Allied Health Program.

Coile, R. C. (1995). Advanced practice nurse: A critical resource for managed care. *Health Trends, 7*(7), 1-7.

Erlen, J., Mellors, M., & Koren, A. (1996). Ethical issues and the new staff mix. *Orthopaedic Nursing, 15*(2), 73-77.

Eriksen, L., Quandt, B., Teinert, D., Look, D., Loosie, R., Mackey, G., & Strout, B. (1992). A registered nurse-licensed vocational nurse partnership model for critical care nursing. *Journal of Nursing Administration, 22*(12), 28-38.

Esselman, C. (1995). Developing a healthcare technician training course. *Nursing Management, 26*(6), 46, 48.

Freidman, E. (1990). Nursing: New power, old problems. *Journal of the American Medical Association, 264*(23), 2977-2982.

Gordon, S. (1997, February). What nurses stand for. *Atlantic Monthly, 279,* 80-88.

Grillo-Peck, A., & Risner, P. (1995). The effect of a partnership model on quality and length of stay. *Nursing Economics, 13*(6), 367-374.

Hansten, R. I., & Washburn, M. J. (1997). Successful restructuring: Maximizing training dollars. *Nursing Economics, 15*(2), 81-86.

Hayes, P. (1994). Non-nursing functions: Time for them to go. *Nursing Economics, 12*(3), 120-125.

Hendricks, J., & Baume, P. (1997). The pricing of nursing care. *Journal of Advanced Nursing, 25,* 454-462.

Hines, P. (1994). An interview with Moira Kelly. *Nursing Economics, 12*(3), 113-119.

Joel, L. (1994). Restructuring: Under what conditions? *American Journal of Nursing, 96*(3), 7.

Johnson, S. (1995). The right balance. *Dimensions of Critical Care Nursing, 14*(1), 2-3.

Kieltyka, C., Robertson, S., & Behner, K. (1997). A flexible staffing model for patient service associates. *Journal of Nursing Administration, 27*(1), 48-54.

Lyon, J. C. (1993). Models of nursing care delivery and case management: Clarification of terms. *Nursing Economics, 11*(3), 163-169.

MacLeod, J. A., & Sella, S. (1992). One year later; Using role theory to evaluate a new delivery system. *Nursing Forum, 27*(2), 20-29.

Manthey, M. (1990). Definitions and basic elements of a patient care delivery system with an emphasis on primary nursing. In G. G. Mayer, M. J. Madden, & E. Lawrenz (Eds.), *Patient care delivery models* (pp. 201-211). Gaithersburg, MD: Aspen.

Manuel, P., & Alster, K. (1994). Unlicensed personnel: No cure for an ailing health care system. *Nursing & Health Care, 15*(1), 18-21.

Manuel, P., & Sorensen, L. (1995). Changing trends in healthcare: Implications for baccalaureate education, practice, and employment. *Journal of Nursing Education, 34*(6), 248-253.

McKenna, H. P. (1995). Nursing skill mix substitutions and quality of care: An exploration of assumptions from the research literature. *Journal of Advanced Nursing, 21*, 452-459.

National Council of State Boards of Nursing. (1995). *Delegation: Concepts and decision-making process.* Chicago: Author.

Neidlinger, S., Bostrom, J., Stricker, A., Hild, J., & Zhang, J. (1993). Incorporating nursing assistive personnel into a nursing professional practice model. *Journal of Nursing Administration, 23*(3), 29-37.

O'Brien, Y., & Stepura, B. (1992). Designing roles for assistive personnel in a rural hospital. *Journal of Nursing Administration, 22*(10), 34-37.

Oregon Revised Statutes. (1995). *Chapter 678. Nurses: Nursing home administrators.* Retrieved August 4, 1998, from the World Wide Web: http://landru.leg.state.or.us/ors/678.html

Pedersen, A., Hoover, C., & Kisiel, T. (1995). Redesigning a skills mix in the ICU. *Nursing Management, 26*(7), 32J-32P.

Pender, N. (1992). Partnerships: An alternative to rugged individualism. *Nursing Outlook, 40*(96), 248-249.

Russo, J., & Lancaster, D. (1995). Evaluating unlicensed assistive personnel models. *Journal of Nursing Administration, 25*(9), 51-57.

Townsend, M. (1994). Twenty-four hour care teams. *Nursing Management, 25*(6), 62-64.

Chapter

7 Advanced Practice Nurses

Acute-Care Settings

Margaret M. Conger

Who am I then? Tell me first, and then if I like being that person, I'll come up; if not, I'll stay down here till I'm somebody else.

Alice (in Lewis Carroll's *Alice in Wonderland*)

Roles for advanced practice nurses (APNs) are rapidly changing in the emerging paradigm of managed care. For some, such as certified nurse anesthetists, the changes are relatively minor. For others, especially the clinical nurse specialists (CNSs), role changes are dramatic. Considerable controversy surrounds the role the CNS should have in the changing health care environment. For many, the dilemma that Alice faced is very real. Who should this nurse become?

Changes in advanced nursing practice are reflected in the nursing literature by debates on education and appropriate roles and tasks for APNs. Some advocate for an APN who is educated in and capable of managing both nurse practitioner (NP) and CNS functions (Cronenwett 1995;

Dunn, 1997; Fenton & Brykczynski, 1993; Fitzgerald & Wood, 1997; Pinelli, 1997; Porter-O'Grady, 1996; Schroer, 1991). These nurses believe that there will be increased job opportunities, less role confusion, and less confusion in the public mind about advanced practice nursing if these roles are combined.

Other nursing leaders have expressed concern about merging the roles of the CNS and the NP (Brown, 1996; Cukr, 1996; Lyon, 1996; Page & Arena, 1994; Woods, 1997). These nurses question the ability of one person to become expert in both roles. In addition, merging roles could "jeopardize important components of the CNS role" (Redekopp, 1997, p. 90). Woods states that "the temptation to prepare an all singing, all dancing supernurse should be resisted and tempered by the reality of clinical practice" (p. 821). To understand the issues important to developing the role for APNs in acute-care hospitals facing the economic constraints of a capitated environment, each of these roles must be described. Nursing administrators need to think through which of these roles best suits the needs of his or her institution. This information is also needed by baccalaureate nurses who are deciding which APN role to pursue in graduate school. An informed decision-making process seems to be a far better approach than to be in Alice's predicament of not knowing who she is. This chapter will discuss several of the APN roles presently in place and review the practice changes occurring in them related to the managed care paradigm. The emphasis of the chapter will be on the newly emerging role of the acute-care nurse practitioner.

Advanced Practice Nurse Roles in Acute-Care Settings

Advanced practice nurses are defined as those who have developed expert skill in a specialized area of practice, usually though nursing education at the master's level. These APNs must also maintain a clinical practice that involves direct patient care as a portion of the practice. Historically, nurses who practiced beyond the basic level included clinical nurse specialists, nurse practitioners, nurse midwives, and nurse anesthetists. All of these have seen changes in their practice within the acute-care hospital as a result of cost constraints in health care delivery.

Nurse Anesthetist

The nurse anesthetist has been a part of the acute-care hospital for many years. In the early years of anesthesia practice, nurses were the primary providers of anesthesia to surgical patients. Currently there are over 25,000 practicing certified registered nurse anesthetists (CRNAs); nurses are the sole providers of anesthesia in over 70% of rural hospitals in the United States (Garde, 1996). The use of the CRNA is on the increase as managed care organizations seek to find cost-effective ways to deliver safe health care.

For many years, registered nurses seeking certification as a nurse anesthetist completed programs based in hospitals and were certified by examination. This practice, however, is changing. As of 1998, all nurse anesthetist educational programs had to be at the master's level, clearly placing this practice within the advanced practice nurse domain. Along with changes in educational standards, the scope of practice for CRNAs is expanding. Although a considerable portion of nurse anesthetist practice still deals with direct administration of anesthetic agents, the management of patients during surgery and the immediate postoperative period is also within their practice. They are responsible for the management of a patient's fluid balance, including inserting catheters for fluid resuscitation and determining the appropriate type and amount of fluid needed. They also manage the patient's airway, using ventilatory support as necessary. As part of their service, they are involved in the management of postoperative pain, including the prescription and set-up of patient-controlled analgesia pumps. In most states, they are able to prescribe pain management drugs (Garde, 1996). In states in which CRNAs do not have prescribing privileges, they work under protocols developed for pain management.

Many of the tasks involved in the CRNA practice require a high level of technical skill, but the nursing skills of these practitioners are also important. Dlugose (1996) emphasizes that the nursing skills of assessment and interpretation of diagnostic data are also central to this practice. CRNAs working in critical care environments are responsible for constantly assessing a patient's physiological responses during surgery and immediately postoperative. They must be able to determine when changes in the therapeutic regimen need alteration. They must also have excellent communication skills to work effectively with patients and families prior to surgery and during the recovery period. These are times of high stress for patients, and the therapeutic communication skills CRNAs acquired during nursing education are vital to their practice. Thus, although the CRNA provides a service within the medical realm, he or she also remains firmly planted within the discipline of nursing.

The future for CRNA practice in the managed care environment is shifting. Faut-Callahan and Kremer (1996) suggest that with the downsizing of acute-care hospitals, the number of CRNAs employed in this setting will decrease. Data from 1994 show that 41% of CRNAs were employed by hospitals, 34% were involved in a group practice arrangement, 12% were self-employed, and 13% were in other types of practice (Faut-Callahan & Kremer, 1996). Another challenge to this practice is the emerging practice of anesthesia assistants, who provide anesthesia services under physician supervision. It may well be that more CRNAs may find employment in outpatient surgical centers if the trend in acute-care hospitals is to employ such providers.

Nurse Midwife

The role of the nurse midwife began as a community role, particularly with populations in rural or inner-city areas who were medically underserved. A philosophical tenet of nurse midwifery practice is the independent management of the childbearing family (Scupholme, DeJoseph, Strobino, & Paine, 1992). As the managed care era grows, more nurse midwives are finding employment within the acute-care hospital setting rather than in independent practice. Others are seeking admitting privileges at hospitals so that they can manage their patients during the labor and delivery period within the hospital setting. A survey conducted by the American College of Nurse-Midwives in 1963 showed that 31% of the nurse midwives reported that they were engaged in clinical practice within a hospital setting (Runnerstrom et al., 1983). This number had increased to 72% by 1991 (Scupholme et al., 1992). Another change reported in this study is of an increasing trend for hospital-employed nurse midwives to attend only the labor and delivery of the woman, with no part in prenatal care (Walsh & DeJoseph, 1993). The American College of Nurse-Midwives data from 1991 (Walsh & DeJoseph, 1993) indicate that 28.3% of those reporting were employed by a hospital, and 7.1% were employed by a health maintenance organization (HMO). Data from a 1997 survey (Kraus, 1997) indicated that 27% were employed by a hospital and 9% were employed by an HMO. Nurse midwife practice within a physician practice also remained fairly constant. In 1991, the percentage of nurse midwives reporting being a part of a physician practice was 25.9%; in 1997 the percentage was 24%. These data suggest that practice patterns for nurse midwives have not changed much over the 8-year period of rapid growth of managed care organizations.

Admitting privileges for certified nurse midwives (CNMs) in acute-care hospitals have been relatively recent. The Washington, D.C. District Council passed legislation in 1983 that provided for nurse midwife practice in obstetrical deliveries within the hospital. At the time, this legislation was considered to provide the broadest practice privileges in the nation (Langton & Kammerer, 1989). It allowed CNMs to obtain privileges to admit patients to the hospital, deliver babies in the obstetrical suite, and follow their patients throughout the hospital stay. The degree of supervision by a physician would be established by each individual hospital. The law stated that the CNM only needed to collaborate with a physician; the degree of this collaboration was left unspecified.

Another model for nurse midwifery practice in acute-care hospitals is as an employee who functions in a birthing center to manage the labor and delivery experience of women considered to be at low risk for obstetrical complications. An example of this model is the Normal Birth Center at Los Angeles County–University of Southern California (Greulich et al., 1994). The center is staffed by CNMs, with at least two present in the unit at all times. Women who are determined to be at low risk for obstetrical complications are admitted to this unit rather than to the high-risk labor and delivery unit. The nurse midwives in this unit do not see the women prior to their onset of labor; instead, the women are managed in community-based clinics and are referred to the Birthing Center only for the delivery.

In addition to the CNMs, the Birthing Center also employs two pediatric nurse practitioners to manage the care of the newborns. The hospital provides around-the-clock physician backup coverage, with both obstetrical and pediatric residents, who can be summoned to the unit as needed. If a woman develops problems during the labor experience, she can be rapidly transferred to the high-risk unit because of the close proximity of the units. In over 10 years of experience in this nurse midwife-staffed unit, the rate of complicated obstetrical deliveries requiring some type of surgical intervention has remained low, around 4% (Greulich et al., 1994). This low rate supports the efficacy of the use of nurse midwives to manage deliveries of low-risk obstetrical patients.

A question that arises from a model such as this is how the values of nurse midwifery that espouse a holistic approach to the management of the childbearing family can be actualized in this type of setting. Lessons from practice have also shown that a client is more apt to sue a practitioner who is not known as compared to one who has established a relationship with the client. Nurse midwives will need to think through practice situations in which there is not an opportunity for relationship building. Consideration of these issues is vital because health care organizations seeking ways to manage costs more efficiently could well push to emulate such models.

Clinical Nurse Specialist

An advanced practice role under considerable scrutiny is that of the clinical nurse specialist (CNS). The changing goals of the managed health care environment have resulted in a decrease in job opportunities for these nurses. The prevailing value under the fee-for-service era was the provision of treatment for illness with maximum use of technology. The question asked in this era was, What is the best management for this catastrophic episode of illness (Roberts-DeGennaro, 1993)? This environment promoted the use of the CNS because of the nursing staff's need for guidance in providing expert care for the patient. In the managed care era, however, there is increased emphasis on managing costs and providing care that is outcome based; the CNS is not seen as an important contributor in this new delivery system.

The traditional role of the CNS includes the components of expert clinical practice, consultation, education, and research. In these roles, the CNS served as a leader in developing nursing as a profession. In some CNS models, responsibility for administrative functions has been added. Haddock (1997) suggests that during the 1980s, many CNSs moved beyond the original CNS roles to incorporate more managerial skills into their practice. Some of these administrative functions were staffing, scheduling, and staff performance appraisals. Other skills included the application of systems theory to organizational practice, administrative decision making, and an emphasis on cost accounting. Other skills more recently added are those needed to conduct quality outcomes management (Cronenwett, 1995; Page & Arena, 1994). With responsibilities in these areas, the focus of concern of the CNS moved away from direct patient care, more to the organization as a whole. Haddock (1997) refers to this expanded role as the second-generation CNS.

The CNS traditionally had responsibilities for both direct and indirect client activities. Direct activities occur when interacting with clients or families; indirect activities include the roles of consultant, educator for nursing staff, and researcher (Haddock, 1997; Hamric, 1989). The role of expert clinician has been a pivotal function in CNS practice. Data from studies suggest that the amount of time spent in this activity varies widely. Meisler and Midyette (1994) suggest that 10% of the CNS's time is spent using clinical expertise. Others found a much greater percentage of time reported in this activity. Malone (1986) and Baker (1987) suggest that over 50% of the CNS's time is spent in the expert clinician role. However, this clinical expertise has often been through counseling other nursing staff rather than direct patient interaction. There is increasing pressure on the CNS to have more responsibility for direct patient management, often working under protocols provided by physicians. In this role, the CNS is moving closer to maintaining direct patient care contact.

The role of consultant for the CNS has been primarily an internal role within the employing institution, in which the CNS works with other staff members to solve complex client situations. Some CNSs moved beyond the realm of their home institution to consult on a wider basis. The consultant role has been described as the most difficult for the CNS to develop because it requires others to perceive the CNS as someone with special expertise (Baker, 1987).

The role of educator makes up a large part of CNS practice. The very fact that the CNS holds an advanced degree in nursing gives instant recognition to this role. The CNS has been responsible for the education of patients and their families, hospital staff, nursing students, and even medical house staff, both informally at the patient's bedside and in classroom settings. It is an expert role that most CNSs develop very early in their career. In contrast to the educator role, the researcher role is often the least used CNS role. Nurses disagree as to whether the CNS is expected to generate new information through research or to focus on using existing research.

In light of the ability of CNSs to alter their role in response to organizational needs in the 1980s, it should not be difficult for these nurses to once again respond to societal needs and alter their practice. In response to a changing health care environment and to new opportunities for advanced nursing practice, many clinical nurse specialists have expanded their practice to take on the role of a nurse case manager. The case manager role has been called, by some nurses, the "third generation" of clinical nurse specialists (Haddock, 1997). Considerable pressure exists within acute-care hospitals for the CNS to develop the role of an acute-care nurse practitioner (ACNP). In this role, the ACNP focuses more on the responsibilities formerly provided by medical house staff, whose numbers have decreased in the managed care environment. Haddock (1997) suggests that the CNS should be able to move into either the ACNP or the NCM role, based on the person's interest. There is certainly a need for both. Those CNSs more interested in diagnosis and treatment will be drawn to the ACNP role; others will be attracted to the nurse case manager role. The ACNP role will be discussed in depth in this chapter. The role for the CNS/case manager will be explored in the next chapter.

Acute-Care Nurse Practitioner

The role of the ACNP is rapidly expanding in large teaching hospitals. Changes in medical residency programs have resulted in fewer physicians available to manage patient care (Richmond & Keane, 1992). Residency positions have been decreased because of increased pressure to move physicians into primary care. The number of hours per week that a resident can work has also been reduced. Another reason for the increased use of ACNPs is the need to rapidly move patients through the acute-care hospital. Costs are best managed by coordinating patient care through both the acute phase of an illness and the postdischarge period. Richmond and Keane (1996) argue that this type of coordination is best done by nurses. Nurses have also demonstrated expertise in managing patient and family response to illness. For these reasons, the introduction of the ACNP makes economic sense in the present health care environment.

Practice Settings

Practice settings for ACNPs are as diverse as the institutions that use them. Buchanan and Powers (1996) describe an emergency department that has established a minor emergency area staffed by nurse practitioners to care for clients seeking primary care. In this setting, the ACNP functions in a manner similar to the community-based NP. The earliest use of an NP in an acute-care setting was in neonatal intensive care units (Lott, Polak, Kenyon, & Kenner, 1996). This role evolved from the movement of pediatric physician residents into primary care settings, leaving a gap in coverage in the intensive care unit. Nurse practitioners took over the day-by-day management of these extremely sick babies, who required close monitoring and frequent changes in the intervention plan.

A number of institutions use ACNPs in critical care settings (Alexander, Bourgeois, Goodman, & Higgs, 1996; Callahan, 1996). Savage (1996) describes the development of the ACNP role in the cardiac surgery department at Yale-New Haven Hospital. The reason cited for the addition of this role was the need for someone other than physician residents to care for patients who had undergone procedures such as angiograms or angioplasty. It was believed that this group of patients were generally stable postprocedure and did not provide the type of experience needed to enhance the education of cardiac resident physicians. Because these patients required more medical supervision than could be provided by staff nurses, the ACNP was seen as the appropriate provider for the level of required care.

The ACNP at Yale-New Haven Hospital developed a program in which she contacted the patients prior to their admission to the unit, followed them through the procedure, managed their postprocedure care, and then did post-discharge follow-up. Many of these activities are similar to those of a nurse case manager, but the additional ability to prescribe medications and order diagnostic or therapeutic tests expedited the patient stay in the postprocedure unit.

Callahan (1996) describes a role for the ACNP in a cardiac surgery area at Beth Israel Medical Center in New York City. The role is similar to that at Yale-New Haven Hospital. The ACNP contacts patients prior to their cardiac surgical procedure and provides preprocedure teaching and assessment. As a nurse practitioner, he or she is able to write preoperative orders and schedule preoperative clinical testing. The nurse practitioners in this agency do not become involved during the surgical procedure or during a stay in the intensive care unit but pick up the management of patients when they are transferred to the cardiac step-down unit. There, they coordinate discharge needs with social workers, home care services, physical therapy, or rehabilitation services. They also follow up with patients postdischarge to evaluate response to the treatment management plan.

Another practice area for the ACNP is surgical services. An example of such practice is provided by Hylka and Beschle (1997), who describe the model developed at the Memorial Health Care Center in Worcester, Massachusetts. The ACNP is involved with the patient on a continuum extending from preadmission for surgery through postoperative care. The ACNP is responsible for the presurgical assessment, organizes the preoperative testing, and does preoperative teaching. Some of the ACNPs assist during surgery. Postoperatively, ACNPs manage much of the patient care, using preapproved protocols. They are also involved in wound management procedures such as staple or suture removal. Because the ACNP can provide a nursing perspective to the patient's care as well as some of the medical management, this institution believes that the quality of surgical care has greatly improved.

ACNPs are also used in psychiatric areas to manage the care of clients with emotional problems (Caverly, 1996). These nurses are authorized to prescribe medications related to treatment of psychiatric problems. Because the focus of their education is in the psychiatric realm, they do not prescribe medications related to medical problems. In this way, they differ from many other nurse practitioners who have prescriptive privileges for more general pharmacological management. Psychiatric nurse practitioners (PNPs), when working with severely and persistently mentally ill clients, may use psychotherapy, family therapy, group therapy, and psychopharmacological therapy. They may also provide psychiatric therapy to patients admitted to general hospitals for medical or surgical therapy who are also in need of mental health therapy.

Standards for ACNP Practice

Standards for acute-care nurse practitioner practice were established by the American Nurses Association (1996) in conjunction with the American Association of Critical Care Nurses. These standards provide the domains of practice considered to be within the realm of the ACNP. They include:

Standard I. Assessment: the acute-care nurse practitioner collects patient data.

Standard II. Diagnosis: The acute-care nurse practitioner analyzes the assessment data in determining diagnosis.

Standard III. Outcome identification: The acute-care nurse practitioner identifies expected outcomes individualized to the patient.

Standard IV. Planning: The acute-care nurse practitioner develops a plan of care that prescribes interventions to attain expected outcomes.

Standard V. Implementation: The acute-care nurse practitioner implements the interventions identified in the multidisciplinary plan of care.

Standard VI. Evaluation: The acute-care nurse practitioner evaluates the patient's progress toward attainment of expected outcomes.

ACNP Practice Issues

As ACNP practice is a newly emerging field for nurses, a number of issues need consideration. State laws governing prescriptive privileges for nurse practitioners differ considerably between states. Many states allow for wide prescriptive privileges; others, such as Illinois and Georgia, restrict such practice. Pearson (1998) provides an update of the status of prescribing privileges for nurse practitioners. As of January 1998, 18 states allow full prescriptive privileges, including prescribing controlled substances, without any requirement for physician supervision. These states tend to have high rural populations. Nineteen states provide for nurse practitioner prescribing privileges with some degree of physician involvement. Interestingly, the examples used in this chapter to describe ACNP practice are all from states—Connecticut, Massachusetts, and New York—in which prescriptive privileges require some degree of physician supervision. Twelve states allow for limited prescriptive privileges, excluding controlled substances, for nurse practitioners under physician supervision. With such variation in this practice issue among states, it is apparent why no one model for ACNP practice can serve the needs of all institutions.

The use of protocols to govern patient management is also an issue. In the model described by Callahan (1996), protocols are used extensively to govern practice within a cardiac surgery service. The physicians in this practice also developed standard order sheets. The model described by Hylka and Beschle (1997) in a surgical service also makes extensive use of protocols for the ACNP to use in patient management. Use of such protocols is particularly important in states that do not allow for prescriptive privileges for nurse practitioners. Protocols, however, are less useful in settings in which there is more variety in patient problems. As the patient population becomes more varied, it is difficult to keep the protocols updated to include the most current thinking about specific disease management.

Another issue that must be addressed when developing a practice role for the ACNP is that of relationships with other health care providers. The relationship with nursing staff can cause some difficulties. In the role of manager of patient care, the ACNP has the authority to assess, diagnose, and develop the treatment plan for patients in his or her caseload. If staff nurses are not comfortable with the role of the CNS, they may hesitate to accept the CNS's orders regarding patient care management. Relationships with physicians can also be problematic. The nurse must move from a subordinate position to one of a colleague if effective communication between the two is going to develop. ACNPs must also establish a role that is neither that of traditional nursing nor that of a substitute physician; they should not be viewed simply as a replacement for house officers. Because ACNPs bring a rich nursing background to their practice, their role incorporates many advanced nursing skills such as health promotion and maintenance, excellent interpersonal skills, and a holistic approach to patients. These nursing skills provide an additional richness to care that goes beyond usual medical practice.

Reporting Issues

The issues of who hires and who supervises the ACNP continue to be problematic. In some settings, the ACNP is hired by nursing and reports to nursing administration. In other models, the ACNP is part of a medical practice staff and reports to a physician(s), gaining hospital privileges through the same credentialing process used by physicians. In such a structure, the ACNP has no formalized relationship with nursing and is often viewed as a physician extender (Norsen et al., 1997). In another model, the ACNP is hired by the hospital but reports to a physician. In both of the physician-related models, the ACNP must develop strategies to create links with nursing so that the role does not become based solely on medical practice.

The advantages of a model in which ACNPs report to the physician staff is that their practice will not be limited by nursing administrators who do not understand independent nursing roles (Lott et al., 1996). When the ACNP reports to a medical team, however, it may be more difficult to retain nursing activities in the role. Often the medical team may expect the ACNP to meet the same time frame in patient management as would a house medical officer, thus reducing the time needed for nursing roles such as education, consultation with patients and families, and other holistic activities. Lott et al. (1996) advocate for the ACNP to be placed within the nursing department, with a strong collaborative relationship with the medical staff. As seen in the examples presented earlier in this discussion, current practice seems to be in the direction of the ACNP reporting to the medical staff.

The lack of role models for ACNP practice may contribute to the confusion about what reporting structure is best. At this time, it seems best for reporting issues to be worked out on a case-by-case basis. As both nursing administrators and medical staff become more familiar with this role, these issues will be better understood. Whether the ACNP is employed by nursing or medicine, positive relationships must be developed among both groups. The ACNP, as an advanced practice nurse, is needed to enhance the professional practice of nursing; as a member of the team responsible for the direct management of patient care, the ACNP must develop a collegial relationship with physicians.

Overlap Between CNS and ACNP Roles

The debate over the development of the role of the ACNP as separate from clinical nurse specialist must also be addressed. Should these roles become one? Those who argue for the merger of these roles suggest there are economic benefits to the hiring institution (Porter-O'Grady, 1996), decreased use of educational resources if these APNs are all trained in the same way (O'Flynn, 1996), and increased name recognition and political power (Lynch, 1996). Brown (1996), on the other hand, argues for a "rainbow" of APNs rather than a blending of the colors. She suggests that there are significant differences between the roles of the CNS and the NP that support the need to maintain separate roles.

An argument for not blending these roles is the difficulty of one nurse to be an "expert" in all roles. The NP and the CNS have knowledge areas that overlap but also areas that are quite distinct. An advanced practice nurse who must be an expert NP *and* an expert CNS will be stressed to develop both roles. "Role strain" has been a common problem among CNSs who were supposed to fill the roles of clinical expert, educator, researcher, consultant, and, many times, administrator. Thus good reasons exist to question the ability of any nurse to add to the existing demands of CNS or NP practice the additional demands of another role. As one nurse practitioner recently noted, "It is possible for this combined role NP to be spread too thinly in trying to execute all of the functions of a greatly expanded role" (Breuninger, 1996, p. 14).

A model that has differentiated between roles for the CNS and the ACNP has been developed at the Strong Memorial Hospital in Rochester, New York (Norsen et al., 1997). In this model, the roles for the ACNP have been built on the traditional roles of the CNS, with the additional important component of direct patient care as the foundation for the role. The role consists of five major components:

Direct patient care
Support systems
Education
Research and publication
Professional leadership (Norsen et al., 1997, p. 154).

Managing Patient Care

In the Strong Memorial model (Norsen et al., 1997), a clear distinction has been made between the practice of the ACNP and that of the CNS. The ACNP role in patient care is similar to those already discussed in this chapter, including conducting the patient history and physical assessment, identifying the need for diagnostic testing, and carrying out specialty-specific procedures. The CNS in this setting does not have a direct patient care role but is more focused on systems issues, such as development of clinical pathways or patient outcome measures. The CNS role is centered more in indirect patient management functions.

Support Systems

The role of the CNS in the area of support systems is an extremely important part of the role. The CNS is expected to be the leader in researching and implementing new nursing procedures and the use of new products. The development of protocols specific to the use of these products is also expected. Both the CNS and the ACNP are expected to be leaders in total quality management processes. Collaboration between these disciplines is appropriate because of the need for a total team approach to quality management. The ACNP also participates in strategic planning for the medical service in which he or she is involved. Thus, although the ACNP will spend a small percentage of time in developing expertise in this area, the CNS is expected to spend a large part of his or her time in activities related to the support of systems.

Education

The role of educator for the CNS is very different from the role of educator for the ACNP in the Strong Model (Norsen et al., 1997). The CNS has a very active role in the education of nursing and other hospital staff, both in orientation efforts and in ongoing clinical education. The role for the ACNP in education is more limited to direct patient and family education on a one-to-one basis. It tends to be more informal: at the bedside, as opposed to a classroom presentation.

Research and Publication and Professional Activities

In the area of research and publication, the two APN roles are more similar (Norsen et al., 1997). Both participate in research related to patient care issues. The emphasis each places on this role will vary. The CNS may spend a considerable percentage of time in this area, particularly in the application of research findings to problems related to patient care issues. The ACNP involvement is often less because of the high time demands of direct patient care responsibilities. Both kinds of APN are involved in professional activities, such as participation in seminars, conferences, and professional organizations.

In the model developed for advanced practice nursing at Strong Memorial Hospital (Norsen et al., 1997), a clear differentiation has been made between CNS and ACNP practice. The ACNP has a very active role in the direct management of patient care; the CNS has continued to have a more indirect role in patient management. It will be interesting to see how CNS practice may change as nursing case management becomes a stronger force in this institution.

Conclusions

The era of managed care has brought with it exciting opportunities for nurses with advanced education to develop new roles within hospital settings. It is little wonder that Coile (1995) has seen advanced practice nursing as the growth area within acute-care hospitals. To meet this challenge, nursing must restructure roles for advanced practice nurses and learn to market newly designed roles. The role for the nurse anesthetist and the certified nurse midwife is growing in acute-care hospitals. The economic value of these nurses in a capitated payment health system is no longer questioned.

The issues related to the use of other advanced practice nurses are more complex. Many large teaching hospitals are developing roles for nurse practitioners within the acute-care hospital. As physician education training continues to be shifted into community settings and primary care, the gap left in the hospital could well be filled by these advanced practice nurses.

Many nursing administrators have questioned the economic viability of the traditional CNS role. Direct patient care responsibilities are critical to the survival of all care providers in the managed care environment. Certainly one option for the CNS is to move into direct patient contact by taking on the role of the nurse case manager, with an emphasis on promoting quality patient outcomes in a cost-efficient manner. In the next chapter, this role in an acute-care hospital will be explored in depth.

References

Alexander, M. K., Bourgeois, A., Goodman, L. R., & Higgs, M. (1996). An acute/critical care nurse practitioner program. *Nursing Management, 27*(12), 28-30.

American Nurses Association. (1996). *Standards of clinical practice and scope of practice for the acute care nurse practitioner*. Washington, DC: American Nurses Publishing.

Baker, P. O. (1987). Model activities for clinical nurse specialist role development. *Clinical Nurse Specialist, 1*(3), 119-123.

Breuninger, K. (1996). CNS and NP role merger? *Nurse Practitioner, 21*(11), 12.

Brown, M. A. (1996, August 1). Primary care nurse practitioners: Don't blend the colors in the rainbow of advanced practice nursing. *Online Journal of Issues in Nursing*. Retrieved September 4, 1998, from the World Wide Web: http://www.nursingworld.org

Buchanan, L., & Powers, R. D. (1996). Establishing an NP-staffed minor emergency area. *NPNews, 4*(3), 1, 6-7.

Callahan, M. (1996). The advanced practice nurse in an acute care setting. *Nursing Clinics of North America, 31*(3), 487-493.

Caverly, S. E. (1996). The role of the psychiatric nurse practitioner. *Nursing Clinics of North America, 31*(3), 449-463.

Coile, R. C. (1995). Advanced practice nurse: A critical resource for managed care. *Health Trends, 7*(7), 1-7.

Cronenwett, L. (1995). Molding the future of advanced practice nursing. *Nursing Outlook, 43*(3), 112-118.

Cukr, P. L. (1996, August 1). Viva La Difference: The nation needs both types of advanced practice nurses: Clinical nurse specialists and nurse practitioners. *Online Journal of Issues in Nursing*. Retrieved September 4, 1998, from the World Wide Web: http://www.nursingworld.org

Dlugose, D. (1996). What is nurse anesthesia practice? *Nursing Clinics of North America, 31*(3), 565-566.

Dunn, L. (1997). A literature review of advanced clinical nursing practice in the United States of America. *Journal of Advanced Nursing, 25,* 814-819.

Faut-Callahan, M., & Kremer, M. (1996). The certified registered nurse anesthetist. In A. B. Hamric, J. A. Spross, & C. M. Hanson (Eds.), *Advanced nursing practice: An integrative approach* (pp. 421-444). Philadelphia: Saunders.

Fenton, M., & Brykczynski, K. (1993). Qualitative distinctions and similarities in the practice of clinical nurse specialists and nurse practitioners. *Journal of Professional Nursing, 9*(6), 313-326.

Fitzgerald, S. M., & Wood, S. H. (1997). Advanced practice nursing: Back to the future. *Journal of Gynecology and Neonatal Nursing, 26*(1), 101-107.

Garde, J. F. (1996). The nurse anesthesia profession: A past, present, and future perspective. *Nursing Clinics of North America, 31*(3), 567-580.

Greulich, B., Paine, L., McClain, C., Barger, M. K., Edwards, N., & Paul, R. (1994). Twelve years and more than 30,000 nurse-midwife attended births: The Los Angeles County–University of Southern California Women's Hospital Birth Center experience. *Journal of Nurse-Midwifery, 39*(4), 185-195.

Haddock, K. S. (1997). Clinical nurse specialist. In S. Moorhead & D. Huber (Eds.), *Nursing roles: Evolving or recycled* (pp. 139-149). Thousand Oaks, CA: Sage.

Hamric, A. B. (1989). History and overview of the CNS role. In A. B. Hamric & J. A. Spross (Eds.), *The clinical nurse specialist in theory and practice* (pp. 3-17). Philadelphia: Saunders.

Hylka, S. C., & Beschle, J. C. (1997). The role of advanced practice nurses in surgical services. *Association of Operating Room Nurses Journal, 66*(3), 481-485.

Kraus, N. (1997). Practice profile of members of the American College of Nurse-Midwives. *Journal of Nurse Midwifery, 42*(4), 355-363.

Langton, P. A., & Kammerer, D.A. (1989). Childbearing and women's choice of nurse-midwives in Washington, D.C. hospitals. *Women and Health, 15*(2), 49-65.

Lott, J. W., Polak, J. D., Kenyon, T. B., & Kenner, C. A. (1996). Acute care nurse practitioner. In A. B. Hamric, J. A. Spross, & C. M. Hanson (Eds.), *Advanced nursing practice: An integrative approach* (pp. 351-373). Philadelphia: Saunders.

Lynch, A. M. (1996, August 1). At the crossroads: We must blend the CNS + NP roles. *Online Journal of Issues in Nursing.* Retrieved September 4, 1998, from the World Wide Web: http://www.nursingworld.org

Lyon, B. L. (1996, August 1). Meeting societal needs for CNS competencies: Why the CNS and NP roles should not be blended in master's degree programs. *Online Journal of Issues in Nursing.* Retrieved September 4, 1998, from the World Wide Web: http://www.nursingworld.org

Malone, B. L. (1986). Evaluation of the clinical nurse specialist. *American Journal of Nursing, 86*(12), 1375-1377.

Meisler, N., & Midyette, P. (1994). CNS to case manager: Broadening the scope. *Nursing Management, 25*(11), 44-46.

Norsen, L., Fineout, E., Fitzgerald, D., Horst, D., Knight, R. Kunz, M. E., Lumb, E., Martin, B., Opladen, J., & Schmidt, E. (1997). The acute care nurse practitioner: Innovative practice for the 21st century. In S. Moorhead & D. G. Huber (Eds.), *Nursing roles: Evolving or recycled?* (pp. 150-169). Thousand Oaks, CA: Sage.

O'Flynn, A. L. (1996). The preparation of advanced practice nurses. *Nursing Clinics of North America, 31*(3), 429-437.

Page, N. E., & Arena, D. M. (1994). Re-thinking the merger of the clinical nurse specialist and the nurse practitioner roles. *Image: The Journal of Nursing Scholarship, 26*(4), 315-318.

Pearson, L. J. (1998). Annual update of how each state stands on legislative issues affecting advanced nursing practice. *Nurse Practitioner, 23*(1), 14-16, 19-20, 25-26, 29-33, 39, 43-46, 49-50, 52-54, 57-58, 61-62, 64, 66.

Pinelli, J. M. (1997). The clinical nurse specialist/nurse practitioner: Oxymoron or match made in heaven? *Canadian Journal of Nurse Administration, 10*(1), 85-110.

Porter-O'Grady, T. (1996). Nurses as advanced practitioners and primary care providers. In E. L. Cohen (Ed.), *Nurse case management in the 21st century* (pp. 10-20). St. Louis, MO: Mosby.

Redekopp, M. A. (1997). Clinical nurse specialist role confusion: The need for identity. *Clinical Nurse Specialist, 11*(2), 87-91.

Richmond, T. S., & Keane, A. (1992). The nurse practitioner in tertiary care. *Journal of Nursing Administration, 22*, 11-12.

Richmond, T. S., & Keane, A. (1996). Acute-care nurse practitioners. In J. V. Hickey, R. M. Ouimette, & S. L. Venegoni (Eds.), *Advanced practice nursing* (pp. 316-326). Philadelphia: Lippincott.

Roberts-DeGennaro, M. (1993). Generalist model of case management practice. *Journal of Case Management, 2*(3), 106-111.

Runnerstrom, L., Cramer, B., Fischman, S., Matousek, I., Nissen, C., & Hogan, A. (1983). *Descriptive data: Nurse midwives U.S.A.* New York: American College of Nurse-Midwives.

Savage, K. (1996). "Exactly what we needed": NP makes a difference in Yale Cardiac Unit. *NPNews, 4*(3), 1, 6.

Schroer, K. (1991). Case management: Clinical nurse specialist and nurse practitioner, converging roles. *Clinical Nurse Specialist, 5*(4), 189-194.

Scupholme, A., DeJoseph, J., Strobino, D. M., & Paine, L. L. (1992). Nurse-midwifery care to vulnerable populations: Phase I: Demographic characteristics of the national CNM sample. *Journal of Nurse-Midwifery, 37*(5), 341-347.

Walsh, L. V., & DeJoseph, J. (1993). Findings of the 1991 Annual American College of Nurse-Midwives Membership Survey. *Journal of Nurse-Midwifery, 38*(1), 35-41.

Woods, L. P. (1997). Conceptualizing advanced nursing practice: Curriculum issues to consider in the educational preparation of advanced practice nurses in the UK. *Journal of Advanced Nursing, 25*(4), 820-828.

Chapter

8 Nurse Case Management

Acute-Care Hospital Practice

Margaret M. Conger
JoAnne Woodall

It was going to be one of Rabbit's busy days. As soon as he woke up, he felt important, as if everything depended upon him. It was just the day for Organizing Something.

Winnie the Pooh (A. A. Milne)

Nurse case managers (NCMs) who are employed in acute-care hospitals must often feel like Rabbit. Every day is one for organizing something—or everything. Often it must seem that everything does depend on the coordinating skills of the NCM. Perhaps, just as Rabbit saw himself as "Captainish" when "everybody said 'Yes, Rabbit' and 'No, Rabbit' and waited until he had told them," NCMs must feel the pressure of countless decisions that need to be made daily. Their skill in managing the care of patients with complex needs within the acute-care setting is vital to managed care organizations to meet their dual goals of cost-effectiveness and quality of care. It requires a great deal of expertise to be an effective "Rabbit." This chapter will explore the skills needed for NCMs to be successful in this new role.

The effectiveness of NCMs in helping managed care organizations to achieve cost and quality goals successfully is the driving force behind their increased use. The strategies used by the NCM to achieve organizational goals will be explored in this chapter. Throughout this discussion, case examples from the practice of the authors will be used to illustrate how these strategies are used in actual practice. All names of actual patients have been altered to protect their identity.

The activities of the NCM will be explored by looking at three periods in the hospitalization of a patient. These include the time of admission, throughout the course of the hospitalization, and, finally, the discharge period. In addition, strategies for evaluating NCM activities will be discussed in terms of specific outcomes. These outcomes are related to cost-effective use of resources, quality of care given, and patient-achieved goals that have been mutually determined.

Admission Activities

Appropriate Location of Services

An important function that must occur at the time of admission to the hospital is determining the appropriateness of the admission. In the managed care environment, this is often first evaluated prior to admission by a precertification process using predetermined criteria. The reviewer will determine what is the most appropriate facility: acute-care hospital, skilled nursing, or an outpatient setting based on the level of service required. However, because information provided during the precertification process may be incomplete or misleading, the patient's status must again be reviewed at the time of admission (Powell, 1996). Often sufficient information to make an absolute determination is not known at the time of admission. In this case, a 24-hour observation period may be authorized so that the physician can make a better determination of the patient status. The nurse is very important to this process, as he or she will do an in-depth assessment of the patient situation and provide this information to the physician so that an informed decision can be made. This role has been traditionally carried out by the utilization review nurse, using standard criteria such as the number of treatment modalities needed or invasive diagnostic procedures planned. As the utilization review function is merging with case management, this is a function now often required of the NCM.

The assessment of need for acute hospitalization needs to take into account not only the acuteness of the illness but a determination of whether services could be provided at a lesser level of intensity. An example that illustrates the complexity of making these decisions is Rosa M., a 71-year-old woman admitted to the hospital with terminal liver disease. She had been cared for at home by her husband, who was finding the burden of her care more than he could continue to manage. It was quickly determined that there was no acute treatment management needed, and a lower level of care would be more appropriate. However, there were no beds available in skilled nursing facilities in the area and probably would not be for the next week. The NCM worked with the family to determine what type of support would be needed to return Rosa to her home and be cared for by the family. The equipment needed for her care at home was a hospital bed with an air mattress and home oxygen services. Home health nursing services, including that of a nursing aide to provide daily care, were also arranged. To make the care of Rosa easier for the family, the NCM talked with the physician and obtained an order for a Foley catheter so that the incontinence problem could be better managed. With these support services in place, Rosa returned home on the day following her hospital admission, and her care was managed by the family. She died 7 days later at home with her family present. When one considers that the cost of each day of hospitalization is over $1,000 a day, the savings generated by moving Rosa back to her home were significant.

Identify Need for Case Management

An important part of the NCM role is to rapidly assess newly admitted patients to determine who may be in need of case management services. A number of nurses have developed screening tools that can be used to do a rapid assessment for the need for case management (Jehle, Terry, & Murphy, 1996; A. Summers, personal communication, October 1995). Indicators that were identified from a review of these tools are summarized in Table 8.1. From this list, an NCM can select those indicators that are relevant to the patient population served and develop an institution-specific screening tool.

In all of the screening tools reviewed, age greater than 70 years was a trigger for further investigation of need for case management. Presence of a

TABLE 8.1 Screening Criteria for Determining Need for Case Management Services

Age greater than 70 years
Chronic illness
AIDS
Cancer
Cardiac
Diabetes
Respiratory
Acute-onset illness
Cerebral vascular accident
High-risk pregnancy
Self-care deficits
Mobility
Management of treatment modalities
Psychological issues
Cognitive deficits
Developmental deficits
Limited coping abilities
Sociological issues
Caregiver—elderly
Caregiver—none
Limited financial resources
History of frequent readmissions to
Acute-care hospital
Emergency Department
Outpatient services
Multiple physicians or discipline involvement

chronic illness such as cardiac, respiratory, cancer, or diabetes was also frequently a trigger. A diagnosis of HIV infection or AIDS should also be a trigger for case management because of the known multiple needs these patients will have. In addition to these chronic conditions, the sudden onset of an illness such as a cerebral vascular hemorrhage or a high-risk pregnancy also indicate need for case management. Also, any sudden change in the ability to manage activities of daily living or treatment modalities indicates a need for case management.

Psychosocial issues also need to be evaluated. A person with cognitive or developmental problems is at high risk for need for case management. A history of chronic mental illness also suggests that there will be a need for intense use of health care resources. Social issues related to caregiver issues such as an elderly caregiver or lack of a caregiver or limited financial resources should also trigger investigation of need for case management.

A final common area among these screens for nurse case management intervention is a history of frequent use of health care resources. Frequent admissions to the acute-care hospital or to the emergency department or outpatient clinics is an indicator of the need for case management involvement. Often the nursing staff can alert the case manager about these people because they are often well known to the unit. Jehle et al. (1996) also suggest that if a patient is being followed by multiple physicians or services, case management will be needed. The coordination of care in these situations often becomes very difficult.

An example of a patient meeting many of these screening criteria is Susan B., a Native American woman living in a fairly isolated community on a reservation. She had a history of multiple hospital admissions for out-of-control congestive heart failure. In a 6-month period prior to the institution of nurse case management services, she had been hospitalized five times with a total of 21 bed days. On the suggested screening tool shown in Table 8.1, Susan would be selected for case management because she meets four of the criteria. These include chronic illness, self-care deficits in terms of managing medication administration, lack of a consistent caregiver, and multiple hospital admissions.

Another example is Sarah D., a 26-year-old woman who was admitted to the hospital with a diagnosis of chest pain. The nurses quickly observed that she was very manipulative in terms of demanding pain medications. She also told very inconsistent stories about her prior treatment and became verbally abusive when she did not get the treatment she demanded. Thus, despite her youth, she met the criteria for case management because of her labile emotional status.

Assessment of Needs

In hospitals that have clinical (critical) pathways in place, a part of the initial assessment process by the staff nurse is to determine the appropriate pathway to use in managing the care of the patient. This decision can often be made by the staff nurse who is admitting the patient. Of course, if the patient has multiple complex problems, the NCM should be available to assist in the decision process. A clinical pathway is a tool that outlines the key events that are expected to happen on each day of the hospitalization for a specific condition. Included also are expected outcomes. The plan should be multidisciplinary in nature so that all health care provider services necessary to manage the care of the patient are included.

When a patient has been identified as needing case management services, there is then need for further in-depth assessment (Powell, 1996). The assessment must include a history that focuses on the medical problem as well as how the patient is managing the problem. Some knowledge of the patient's financial status is needed, particularly in terms of resources available to deal with the current illness. The assessment must also include information about the physical environment of the home that will affect the patient's return to that setting. The ability of the patient to carry out activities of daily living such as hygiene, nutrition, and daily household chores must also be assessed. A psychosocial assessment that includes both the patient's and the family's coping mechanisms to manage the health issue must be considered when developing a plan for the patient.

Mutual Goal Setting

A cardinal principle of the managed care environment is to initiate the development of the discharge plan at the time of admission to the acute-care hospital. However, this plan cannot be made in the absence of patient and family input. Wadas (1993) emphasizes that the NCM begins a long-term relationship with a client in the process of beginning to establish mutually agreed-upon goals. It is important to include both the patient and the family in developing a plan for what will occur both while in the acute-care hospital and following discharge. Even in cases in which the patient is too sick to participate in the decision process, it is important to work with the family to try to identify what they believe the patient would want (Powell, 1996).

At times, this can become very difficult because the patient or family may not be ready to face the reality of the health situation. Powell (1996) cites the example of a daughter of a patient with terminal cancer who only wanted to focus on the need for her mother to have some dental work done. She was not yet ready to talk about the need for hospice care. In times like this, the NCM must work with the family to develop a plan that may seem not the best in the

NCM's eyes but is all the family is ready for at this time. However, the astute NCM will have an alternate plan in mind so that when the family is ready to face the realities of the situation, a more appropriate plan can be put in place.

Papenhausen (1996) suggests principles for the NCM to keep in mind when trying to establish mutually agreed-upon goals. The first is that one should always be working to build self-reliance in the patient and family. Because a goal of nurse case management is to assist patients to make informed choices, it is necessary to discuss options available to the patient and explore the alternatives. Because of the type of fiscal reimbursement that the patient has available, not all options that would be desirable may be open to the patient. In these situations, the NCM can either advocate for an option that may not be readily available or work with the family to find an acceptable plan within the available options. At all times, it is vital to the NCM-patient relationship to respect the choices that the patient may make.

In the situation of Rosa M. discussed earlier in this chapter, these principles of mutual goal setting are demonstrated. The family's first plan was to have Rosa admitted to a skilled nursing setting. However, because no skilled nursing beds were available, the NCM worked with the family to explore other options. With adequate support systems in place, the family was able to manage her care at home.

Concurrent Review

Tools Used for Monitoring Patient Progress

An important cost containment strategy of all managed care organizations is to maintain very strict oversight of patient stays within an institutional setting. This oversight is especially important in the acute-care hospital, where costs can escalate very quickly. The way this is managed will vary between organizations, but all will have some system in place to monitor patient progress throughout the hospital stay. Data is collected for aggregate patient populations to discover trends in usage patterns as well as for individual patients' patterns. The usual practice patterns for each case type (that is, patients with the same diagnostic related group [DRG] designation), including the average length of stay, will be identified. Also, data to identify patient problems that commonly occur with each DRG type will be collected and analyzed to predict future cost and usage patterns. Finally, clinical outcomes that are attainable at the end of the entire expected episode of care and the activities needed to achieve these desired outcomes must be identified (Trinidad, 1993). Nurses are often employed by a managed care organization to carry out these data collection activities.

In addition to the activities that center on data collection for aggregate groups, careful monitoring of individual patients through a treatment episode in an acute-care hospital is also needed. For this process, a systematic means is needed to evaluate the care provided. NCMs are often employed directly by the managed care organization for this monitoring process. The NCM may be situated at the managed care organization and remain in telephone contact with the nursing staff at the hospital; he or she may make occasional rounds at the hospital. The NCM may also be situated at the hospital itself if the managed care organization has a high patient volume using that facility.

Increasingly, managed care organizations are using some type of structured care methodology to assist in this data collection process. A structured care methodology is a tool to identify the best practice for a specific case type. Its use helps to standardize practice in a community. It is also a systematic means to evaluate the care provided. Tools that have been commonly used in the past include standards of care, protocols, or algorithms. The newest tool for this use is the clinical pathway (Cole, Lasker-Hertz, Grady, Clark, & Houston, 1996). The clinical pathway has been given a variety of names. Some common names include *critical pathway* (Zander, 1988), *care map* (Del Togno-Armanasco, Hopkins, & Harter, 1995), *care path* (Weilitz & Potter, 1993), *care pathway* (Gibbs, Lonowski, Meyer, & Newlin, 1995), and *clinical pathway* (Powell, 1996).

Despite the name used, the pathway has many commonalities. It provides written criteria developed by a multidisciplinary team that reflects the standard of practice in the community for managing a patient with a specific medical problem such as congestive heart failure or total hip replacement. It will indicate the appropriate treatment for a particular clinical situation, giving expected time frames in which the treatment will be provided. It also provides outcome criteria to use as an evaluation tool. The pathway can also be a place in which the nurse documents care provided and achievement of intermediate goals (Trinidad, 1993). The purpose of the tool is to provide a guide for managing the care of persons within a given population in a cost-efficient and resource-efficient manner. Because the pathway has been developed by an interdisciplinary group, it is expected that the guideline provided will reflect a more holistic approach to patient management than did its predecessor, the nursing care plan.

The clinical pathway can also be used as a tool to measure the quality of care because of the inclusion of specific time frames for events to happen and specific outcomes to be achieved, both at points along the continuum of the stay and at the point of discharge. The process of variance analysis is used in conjunction with the clinical pathway. Either the staff nurse or the case manager reviews the patient's progress on the pathway at least once every 24 hours. If a specific objective or a specific treatment modality is not achieved within the stated time frame, an analysis of what has prevented its completion must be conducted. There may be a need to request consultation from another health care provider to solve the problem. All variances must be reported in the change-of-shift report to identify important issues that the nurse taking over the management of the patient will need to address.

Variance analysis has become an important tool for measuring both cost-effective and quality-of-care issues. Generally, the reason for a variance can be found in one of three areas. The patient or the patient's family may be the reason for variance from the pathway. The patient may have had an unexpected physiological event such as an elevated temperature, an unexpected amount of pain, or refusal of a medication or treatment. The family may refuse to allow a certain laboratory or diagnostic test to be done. There can also be practitioner-caused variances. The practitioner may inadvertently omit doing a test or procedure listed on the pathway. The physician may determine that a particular event is not needed for this specific patient. Another cause may be an error on the part of a practitioner that results in an unexpected patient complication. The third category of variance is that of a system problem. There may be equipment or personnel shortages that preclude reaching the desired objective within the allotted time frame, or there may be a problem of transferring the patient to a lesser acuity care level due to the inavailabilty of a bed. Any system problem that prevents the patient from moving though the events outlined on the pathway needs to be carefully scrutinized. These are often the most readily "fixable" problems and can greatly affect the achievement of cost-efficient and quality goals desired in the managed care environment. A more in-depth discussion of the legal and ethical implications of the use of the clinical pathway system will be presented in the next chapter.

Variance identification is important to the total quality management/continuous quality improvement (TQM/CQI) process as well as to direct patient monitoring. The outcomes identified on the clinical pathway are used as benchmarks for the TQM/CQI process. An acceptable range for compliance for each outcome on the pathway is determined by a multidisciplinary quality management team. Variances are reviewed at regular established intervals and those that suggest possible problem areas are investigated. It must be emphasized that the process of monitoring variance analysis is not to be used as a "witchhunt" to make particular individuals or departments appear incompetent. Its purpose is to identify areas where problems exist and find creative solutions to improve the quality of care.

An example that demonstrates this process is helpful in making these points. An outcome on the pathway used to manage patients following a mastectomy is that a referral to the Reach for Recovery, a postmastectomy support group, should be provided to all patients prior to discharge. It was found on review of variance analysis that less than 50% of the patients were receiving this referral. The low rate of referral was seen as a problem that could significantly reduce positive patient outcomes.

To address this issue, a study is currently underway to identify the best time for the Reach for Recovery referral to be made. With the very short postsurgical hospital stay following mastectomy that is current practice, many nurses report that the patient is not ready for coping with postsurgical issues during the hospital stay. The patient's attention is on pain management, wound issues, and other postoperative problems. An alternate time seems to be needed to work with these patients on long-term recovery issues. Thus, consideration is being given either to providing the referral about the support group during the presurgical teaching, often in the physician's office, or to developing a more aggressive postdischarge follow-up program. The NCM working with the mastectomy group is currently interviewing women 6 months to 1 year postmastectomy to obtain their opinions on how best to handle this referral.

Monitoring Activities

The person who will be responsible for monitoring the patient's progress throughout the hospital stay varies among organizations. The nurse case manager is often charged with this responsibility. However, it is probably not realistic to expect that there will be sufficient nurse case managers to monitor all patients' care. In practice, a pattern that is commonly seen is for the nurse case manager to quickly screen all new admissions to the nursing unit and identify those who meet the criteria for being at high risk for complex care. If the patient is evaluated as having no high-risk needs, the staff nurse assumes responsibility for the management of that patient's care; the NCM may only become involved to the point of making sure that the appropriate clinical pathway has been instituted. The NCM role in this situation is to be a support person for the nursing staff. Also, the expertise of NCMs is needed in developing the protocols and pathways for use with high-volume, high-risk patient conditions. As these tools are developed, these patients may then be managed by the staff nurse even though the care required may be complex.

Care Management

As long as a patient is moving though the expected course of stay, it is not necessary for the NCM to be involved in the day-by-day monitoring process. Staff nurses thus can monitor the care of patients who fall within the expected guidelines through the use of clinical pathways. With these two levels of patient monitoring, there has been confusion about the terms *case manager* and *care manager*. Ignaviticius (1996) suggests that the nurse who is providing direct bedside care or is supervising a nurse extender at the bedside is providing care management. This includes the day-by-day management of care of patients who do not meet the criteria for specialized case management. The accountability of the care manager is that of monitoring progress using the clinical pathway as a guide. But care management does not provide for the total accountability of the patient's episode of illness as does case management.

Mahn and Spross (1996) also differentiate between the role of the care manager and that of the case manager. They suggest that differentiating factors should be based on patient complexity and predictability of the clinical course. If the clinical situation is simple or common, time limited, predictable, and requires few or inexpensive resources, a staff nurse using a pathway can easily manage the situation. The NCM's expertise is required when the patient situation is very complex, resource intensive, or unpredictable. These differences between care management and case management are depicted in Figures 8.1, 8.2, and 8.3. For a patient who has a well-defined problem such as congestive heart failure with no other complicating features, the clinical pathway is adequate to provide guidance for appropriate care. The relationship

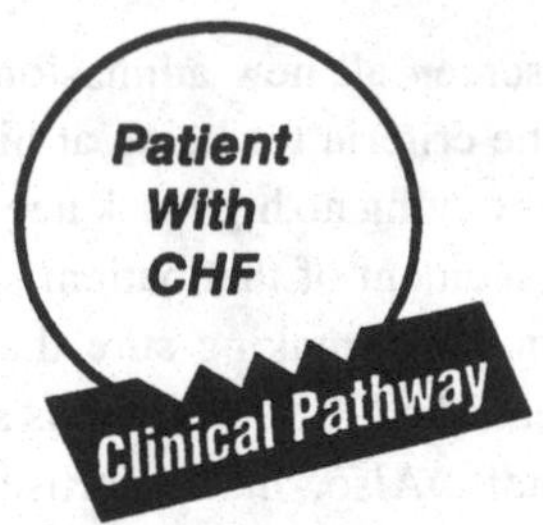

Figure 8.1 Relationship of Patient With Well-Defined Problem and Clinical Pathway

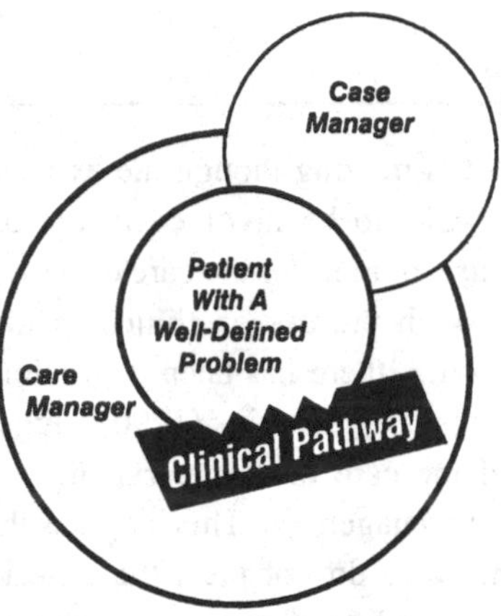

Figure 8.2 Relationship Between Care Manager and Case Manager With Patient With Well-Defined Problem

between the problem and the clinical pathway is depicted in Figure 8.1. For a patient whose care falls within the guidelines of a clinical pathway, the staff nurse can function as the care manager, with limited consultation with the nurse case manager. This is shown in Figure 8.2. However, for those patients who have multiple problems that lie beyond the scope of a clinical pathway, the skills of the nurse case manager are needed. The case manager will focus on developing solutions for those problems that lie beyond the scope of the pathway. This relationship is shown in Figure 8.3. The examples presented in this chapter illustrate a variety of complex problems that require case manager expertise. In these situations, the care manager (staff nurse) and the case

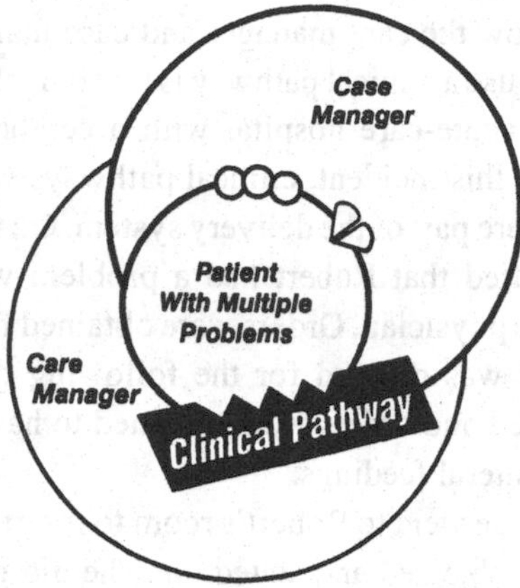

Figure 8.3 Relationship Between Care Manager and Case Manager With a Patient With Multiple Problems

manager need to work collaboratively to assist the patient to achieve optimal outcomes.

There is also a difference between the care manager and the case manager in terms of accountability. Care management is limited to one geographical setting; case management moves across the traditional boundaries of service delivery centers. This broader accountability is what differentiates the practice of the care manager and the case manager. All RNs are now expected to be care managers, with a focus on the client and coordinating care. Nursing case management moves beyond. Roberts-DeGennaro (1993) suggests that the depth needed in each of these functions is what differentiates the case manager from the staff nurse. Each institution will need to work through these issues and determine what the appropriate mix is of baccalaureate-prepared care managers and advanced practice nurse case managers. The end goal in this decision process will be how best to meet the institution's quality and cost-effectiveness goals.

Another trigger for identifying the need for NCM involvement is a pattern of deviation, or variance, from the clinical pathway. It seems reasonable to expect that if a care manager finds that the patient is experiencing a number of variances that will prevent him or her from reaching the desired outcomes, consultation with the nurse case manager is needed. There could well be issues that will need the more in-depth guidance of the NCM.

An example of how the care manager and case manager could function together effectively to use a clinical pathway is that of Robert H., a 72-year-old man admitted to the acute-care hospital with a cerebral vascular accident (CVA). At the time of this incident, clinical pathways were not in use in the hospital, but NCMs were part of the delivery system. On the day of admission, the staff nurse identified that Robert had a problem with swallowing and discussed this with the physician. Orders were obtained for an NPO status and a swallowing consult was ordered for the following day. The swallowing problem was confirmed and orders were obtained to have a nasogastric tube inserted and to start enteral feedings.

When the staff nurse went to Robert's room to insert the nasogastric tube, Claire, Robert's wife, objected and stated that she did not want "any tubes" for Robert. Robert was not able to give a coherent response at that time and was not consulted in the decision. Claire's objection to the feeding tube was not discussed further and no action was taken. Robert remained NPO for one week with no further attempts to provide nutritional support. At that time, he was taken to surgery for placement of a gastric tube and enteral feedings were started. However, after a week of no nutritional support, Robert did not tolerate the feedings well and had a very difficult 2-day period in which the progression of his enteral feedings was very slow. The course of his acute-care hospital stay was finally 9 days, far longer than is expected for a diagnosis of CVA under the prospective payment plan. The general guideline for a hospital stay for a person with a CVA is 6.7 days under the Medicare DRG prospective payment plan (Federal Register, 1993).

Now consider this same scenario if a clinical pathway and variance analysis had been in place. On Day 2, when the enteral feeding was not started, a variance would have been noted on the pathway. If the staff nurse—the care manager—had not been able to negotiate with Claire to solve the problem, a referral to the NCM could have been made. With the advanced negotiation skills of the NCM, a more rapid resolution to the problem would have most likely been found. Exploring her objection to the nasogastric tube with Claire and educating her about the need for nutrition would have been helpful. The identification of the lack of nutrition as a variance from the pathway would have alerted all of the providers of the need for problem resolution. In doing so, Robert's care could have been provided in a far more cost-efficient manner, and at the same time quality of care could have been improved. The surgery for insertion of a gastric tube could most likely have been avoided and Robert could have been moved into a rehabilitation program faster. Thus, the use of the pathway with variance analysis methods could have met the desired goals of health care: efficient use of resources provided in a quality manner.

Functions of the Nurse Case Manager During the Hospital Stay

The role of the nurse case manager in managing patient stays in the acute-care setting includes the overall development of care needs, coordination of multiple services, and follow-up as the patient moves from one care setting within the hospital into other settings in the community. The accountability for the patient is long term and moves beyond the immediate care unit. To carry out these responsibilities, a number of strategies are commonly used by NCMs.

Care Conferences

Many of the patients that are part of the NCM caseload in the acute-care hospital have clinical problems that are difficult to resolve. When a patient is identified as one who will have a long and complicated hospital course, the use of a care conference can be helpful. The conference should include all of the providers caring for the patient, the patient and family, and the NCM. An example that illustrates this activity is that of Henry, a patient who had a number of postoperative complications following gall bladder surgery. During his hospitalization, he had nine surgical procedures and a number of medical complications, including septicemia, septic shock, renal insufficiency, and pancreatic inflammation. An ongoing problem for this man was to find a means to maintain his nutritional status despite the number of gastrointestinal complications. His care team included nine physicians as well as a host of other health care providers. His family consisted of his wife, who lived about 90 miles from the hospital, and a daughter, who lived in an adjoining state and was only able to be at the hospital about 3 days each week. With a complicated hospitalization such as this, it was difficult to get agreement on a plan of care and then to communicate this care to the family. The daughter perceived that the care was fragmented and became angry about what she saw as inadequate care from the nursing staff and the physicians.

The nurse case manager was asked to take over the coordination of this patient's care and to work with the daughter to keep her informed as to what was happening. Through careful explanations, some of the daughter's anger was diffused. At one point, Henry was experiencing a problem with his nutritional feedings and appeared to be regressing. The NCM called a conference with the primary physician, the gastroenterologist, the nutritionist, and the family. The outcome of the conference was to develop a plan to get Henry restarted on his enteral feedings. The inclusion of the entire team was important to this decision. Also, including the family in the conference made it possible for their wishes to be articulated to the physicians. In this situation, the interventions of the NCM were successful in moving Henry through this very difficult period. They also resulted in getting him ready for movement to a skilled nursing facility more rapidly than if no one had been there at critical points to get the plan of care revised.

Collaboration

Another important component of the NCM role is the need to collaborate with multiple health care providers to coordinate services so that the client moves through the health care system in a cost- and time-efficient manner. An example that illustrates this function is a young man, Gabriel, who was admitted to the hospital with abdominal pain. Further diagnostic testing revealed multiple diagnoses, including extrapulmonary tuberculosis and AIDS. In addition to these serious medical problems, Gabriel had a number of social problems that further complicated his situation. He had no health insurance and was unemployed. He was unable to prove his United States citizenship status at the time of his hospital admission and thus was unable to qualify for the Medicaid program.

To obtain services needed for Gabriel, the NCM had to coordinate with a number of agencies. She contacted the county in which he said he was born and was able to obtain a birth certificate proving his citizenship. This then made him eligible to qualify for health care under the Medicaid program. Referrals were made to the county health department for follow-up with his family and neighborhood contacts for evaluation for tuberculosis exposure. A referral was made to the local AIDS organization and a Spanish-speaking AIDS educator was secured to talk with him. A home health visit on the evening of his discharge from the hospital was arranged to make sure he was taking his medications as ordered. This example illustrates that when patients have multiple health care and social problems such as Gabriel, the coordination with a number of other services is an essential part of the care. This complex management goes beyond the scope of the normal clinical pathway and thus needs the interventions of an experienced NCM.

Patient Advocacy

The examples of both Gabriel and Henry illustrate how the NCM functions as a patient advocate. Another example of how the NCM functions as a patient advocate is that of Alice, an elderly woman dying of advanced liver failure and renal insufficiency. Alice had been a patient well known to the hospital through her course of illness. She returned with an intracranial bleed that led to severe neurological deficits that appeared to preclude her ability to return home. It was determined that Alice would need nursing home care but had no health insurance that would pay for this service. The NCM was able to negotiate with the insurance company to transfer some of the benefits provided for hospice care under the insurance policy to cover the cost of the nursing home care. In this way, the patient was able to be moved out of the expensive acute-care setting into less costly care. The role of the NCM as the patient advocate in this situation ensured both a reduction in cost of care and the provision of high-quality care. Without the advocacy of the experienced case manager, it is unlikely that the family would have been able to work through the "system" to achieve a mutually satisfying solution to the problem.

Negotiator

Another role of the NCM is that of negotiator. This negotiation may be with patients, their family members, other members of the health care team, or the third-party payor. An example that illustrates the need for negotiation is that of Jane, a 58-year-old university professor dying from metastatic breast cancer. Jane's mother had come to be with her daughter and was not prepared for her terminal condition. She was still hopeful that continued chemotherapy would bring improvement and that Jane would be able to return home.

Jane's mother was very concerned about the treatment plan, which would provide only comfort measures that could be managed in a skilled nursing facility. The NCM explored with her a number of options, such as home health nursing, hospice care, and skilled nursing care. It soon became apparent that the mother was unable to provide the necessary physical care that Jane needed, even with the assistance of home health nurses and a number of friends. Thus, returning home was not a possibility. To carry out the transfer to the skilled nursing facility, the NCM took Jane's mother over to the facility, introduced her to the staff, and toured the unit until the mother felt comfortable with the level of care provided there. With this type of interaction between the NCM and Jane's mother, approval for the transfer was obtained and care was provided at a lower cost. However, this was achieved only through the excellent negotiation skills of the NCM.

Culturally Appropriate Care

Because the responsibilities of an NCM must encompass the care of patients coming from diverse backgrounds, there is a need to understand and use culturally appropriate interventions. The NCM must undergo a developmental process that includes self-awareness and understanding of others within their cultural reference. The NCM must also acquire the skills needed to provide this culturally relevant and culturally sensitive practice (Rogers, 1995). The following example demonstrates such practice. Ben Y., a 60-year-old Native American man, was hospitalized with an active gastrointestinal bleed. His condition had progressed to that of terminal, with no urine output, rapidly falling blood pressure, and no response to most stimuli. However, he had a full code status, with the family expecting all possible treatments to be provided. This situation is very difficult with some Native American patients because of a cultural belief that if you talk about the possibility of death, you are causing death. Thus, if the family agreed to a no code status, this could be construed as willing the person's death. This situation then required great cultural sensitivity. The family was approached and agreement was reached to take no extraordinary measures to prolong life. The outcome of this situation was that Ben died several hours later with a peaceful death, and the family was supported throughout the process.

Discharge Process

Discharge Planning: Managing Transitions Through the System

In all of these examples, the role of the NCM in managing transitions from one setting to another has been seen. The time of transition is often one in which the NCM must exert much effort. The discharge plan must be started early in the course of the hospitalization, and the amount of attention to it will increase as the time for discharge comes closer. With the use of a clinical pathway, this time should be somewhat predictable. If the patient has been on target with the outcomes on the plan and has had few variances, the time of discharge should be well established.

Some of the discharge services that the patient will need must be planned for early in the course of the patient's stay. Examples of these include arrangements for transfer to a less-acute setting such as a skilled nursing or rehabilitation center. Often it takes several days for a bed in such a facility to become available. It is better to have a reservation for the bed in place early and then have to delay transfer than to have to keep the patient in the acute-care hospital for several extra days while waiting for a placement (Powell, 1996). Anders (1993) found that one of the most frequent reasons for delay in discharge in his community (Hawaii) was the lack of beds in a skilled nursing facility.

Powell (1996) provides a list of activities that the NCM must attend to on the day prior to the expected discharge to make sure that the transfer will go smoothly. Any equipment that needs to be in place when the patient returns home should be checked on. This includes such items as oxygen equipment, special beds, a wheelchair, or special medications. If the services of a home health nurse, physical therapist, respiratory therapist, or other health care provider will be needed to assist the patient in making a smooth transition, the arrangement for these should be rechecked the day prior to discharge. Transportation needs should also be checked on. If special transportation such as a medical van or an air flight to an out-of-state location is needed, these arrangements also need to rechecked the day prior to the expected discharge.

The stability of the patient also needs to be evaluated on the day prior to the expected discharge. Any lab tests that will be needed to evaluate the patient's readiness for discharge should be ordered. Also, teaching needs for both the family and the patient should be verified as completed. The practice of trying to do discharge teaching as the patient's transportation is standing by is not an acceptable practice. At this time, it is also a good idea to provide the patient or family member with a list of postdischarge appointments for follow-up care and review this information to make sure that it is understood. Prescriptions for medications that will be needed at home should also be prepared in advance so that the family can get the needed medications while pharmacies in the community are open. A late evening or weekend discharge can produce problems in this area.

The role of the NCM in the discharge process is extremely important. Often the ability of the family to cope with ongoing care is directly correlated with the thoroughness of the discharge preparation. If all of the needed services are available when the patient reaches home, the family will be empowered to carry out the treatment needs at home.

Following the actual discharge of the patient, the work of the NCM is not finished. Evaluation of how the discharge plan is working is needed. However, there is a great deal of variation between different models of case management at this point. Some hospital models will use a telephone call for follow-up to evaluate the success of the discharge. The call may be made directly to the patient or family or to an out-of-hospital case manager who will continue to follow the client (Brockopp, Porter, Kinnaird, & Silberman, 1992; Zander, 1988). Some models use home visits or meet the client in the clinic setting (Gibbs et al., 1995; Mahn, 1993). A problem that NCMs working within the hospital must face is one of time. It is not always possible to do effective follow-up of patients who have returned to the community because of problems with managing the case load of hospitalized patients. When out of the hospital making the home visits, the NCM may miss the opportunity to speak with a physician about another patient or to work with a family that may be at the hospital for only a short time. Another problem is that the nurse who has been socialized into the acute-care setting may have difficulty moving into the home setting without extensive in-service preparation. Thus, in the Carondelet St. Mary's system, as in others, the in-hospital case manager has pulled back from spending a great deal of time in the community and has rather focused on improving the communication process with other out-of-hospital case managers to ensure that the discharge plan will be accomplished (More & Mandell, 1997).

This final stage of case management—postdischarge evaluation—is extremely important. Often questions arise about the client's care that were not anticipated while the client was still in the hospital. Sometimes problems arise with obtaining the equipment or medications needed. Some clients will need additional encouragement to make contact with support groups, such as Reach to Recovery for postmastectomy patients. A small amount of reassurance and problem solving at this point may make the transition to home successful and thus prevent readmission to the hospital because the family cannot cope with the problems encountered.

Several of the case examples used in this chapter illustrate the importance of the discharge planning and follow-up. Gabriel, the young man with TB and AIDS, required a number of services to manage his discharge to home safely. The NCM arranged for a home health visit the evening of his hospital discharge to ensure that he was taking medications as ordered. With an infectious disease, this is a particularly important element of the treatment plan. Rosa, the woman dying from liver disease, is another excellent example of the need for intense discharge planning. She needed not only a number of pieces of medical equipment but also the services of a variety of professionals. It was only when an extensive discharge plan was in place that her family was able to take her back home, where she died with her family at her side.

Conclusions

The role of the NCM in the hospital setting is demanding but very rewarding. During the course of the patient's stay, many perplexing problems arise. Yet, with the presence of a skilled NCM, answers can be found to meet the needs of both the patient and the organization. With the demands for shorter, more efficient hospital stays in the managed care environment, the skills of the NCM will be tested to the extreme. Yet, when one looks back at a patient episode and can see that the efforts expended resulted in improved quality of life (or death) for the patient and the family needs have been addressed, it is an extremely satisfying role. Perhaps it is professional nursing being demonstrated in its finest expression.

References

Anders, R. L. (1993). Administrative delays: Is there a difference between for-profit and non-profit hospitals? *Journal of Nursing Administration, 23*(11), 42-50.

Brockopp, D. Y., Porter, M., Kinnaird, S., & Silberman, S. (1992). Fiscal and clinical evaluation of patient care. *Journal of Nursing Administration, 22*(9), 23-27.

Cole, L., Lasker-Hertz, S., Grady, G., Clark, M., & Houston, S. (1996). Structured care methodologies: Tools for standardization and outcome measurements. *Nursing Case Management, 1*(4), 160-172.

Del Togno-Armanasco, V., Hopkins, L. A., & Harter, S. (1995). How case management really works. *American Journal of Nursing, 95*(5), 241-24L.

Federal Register. (1993, September 1). *Rules and regulations,* 58(168), 42 CFR Parts 412 & 413 RIN 0938-AG23, p. 46390.

Gibbs, B., Lonowski, L., Meyer, P. J., & Newlin, P. J. (1995). The role of the clinical nurse specialist and the nurse manager in case management. *Journal of Nursing Administration, 25*(5), 28-34.

Ignaviticius, D. (1996, August). *Managed care: Nursing responses.* Paper presented at the Seventh Annual Nurse Educators Conference in the Rockies, Copper Mountain, CO.

Jehle, S., Terry, G., & Murphy, M. (1996). Implementing nurse case management in a rural community hospital. In E. L. Cohen (Ed.), *Nurse case management in the 21st century* (pp. 211-221). St. Louis, MO: Mosby.

Mahn, V. (1993). Clinical nurse case management: A service line approach. *Nursing Management, 24*(9), 48-50.

Mahn, V. A., & Spross, J. A. (1996). Nurse case management as an advanced practice role. In A. B. Hamric, J. A. Spross, & C. M. Hanson (Eds.), *Advanced nursing practice: An integrative approach* (pp. 445-465). Philadelphia: Saunders.

More, P. K., & Mandell, S. (1997). *Nursing case management: An evolving practice.* New York: McGraw-Hill.

Papenhausen, J. L. (1996). Discovering and achieving client outcomes. In E. L. Cohen (Ed.), *Nurse case management in the 21st century* (pp. 257-268). St. Louis, MO: Mosby.

Powell, S. K. (1996). *Nursing case management: A practical guide to success in managed care.* Philadelphia: Lippincott-Raven.

Roberts-DeGennaro, M. (1993). Generalist model of case management practice. *Journal of Case Management, 2*(3), 106-111.

Rogers, G. (1995). Educating case managers for culturally competent practice. *Journal of Case Management, 4*(2), 60-65.

Trinidad, E. (1993). Case management: A model of CNS practice. *Clinical Nurse Specialist, 7*(4), 221-223.

Wadas, T. M. (1993). Case management and caring behavior. *Nursing Management, 24*(9), 40-45.

Weilitz, P. B., & Potter, P. A. (1993). A managed care system: Financial and clinical evaluation. *Journal of Nursing Administration, 23*(11), 51-57.

Zander, K. (1988). Nursing case management: Strategic management of cost and quality outcomes. *Journal of Nursing Administration, 18*(5), 23-30.

Chapter

9

Automated Clinical Pathways in the Patient Record

Legal Implications

Lisa Brugh

Nurses have long been taught the need for precise documentation of patient care. The statement, "If it is not documented, it is presumed not done" is commonly made to beginning nurses, as well as new staff nurses. Yet, as demands on the nurse's time increase, maintaining an accurate and informative patient record becomes more difficult. New methods are needed to address this issue. The use of a patient chart that is maintained on a computer containing both the plan of care and a record of the care is a promising solution to the problem. A clinical pathway that outlines patient care is being used as a place in which the various disciplines document the care given to patients and the patient's progress towards goals and outcomes. When this pathway is a computer-generated form, communication between nurses, physicians, and other care providers is enhanced. The use of a computer-based clinical pathway is an exciting innovation in patient care delivery.

Clinical pathways are being used across the country as hospitals restructure to streamline care while increasing quality and efficiency. The clinical pathway is the tool used to coordinate the time-dependent progress of a typical uncomplicated patient across many clinical departments. The pathway is designed to be specific for the condition or disease being managed (Spooner & Yockey, 1996). Hospitals are using clinical pathways to promote interdisciplinary and outcome-focused care and to reduce professional boundaries and departmental competition. The use of clinical pathways has also provided caregivers with a common language, enhanced accountability, and interdisciplinary ownership (Bultema, Mailliard, Getzfrid, Lerner, & Colone, 1996).

When a clinical pathway becomes a permanent part of a patient's record, the issue of legal liability is questioned. What is a provider's liability in malpractice litigation when the pathway is used as a standard of care (Cole, Lasker-Hertz, Grady, Clark, & Houston, 1996)? Another question is whether or not the potential for malpractice litigation is increased when the pathway, with its documentation, is retained as part of the permanent record. These issues are yet to be tried in the court system.

In this chapter, the development of a pathway and its use in a computerized format as documentation, a record used by all care providers, will be discussed. Issues related to its status as a permanent part of the patient's record will also be considered. The legal implications of the pathway as a standard of care will also be examined.

The Clinical Pathway

The clinical pathway is replacing the traditional nursing care plan. Clinical pathways tie individual care plans of specialized groups into a "team plan," which provides a system that can increase efficiency, promote quality care, and ultimately save the health care system time and money (Kirton, Civetta, & Hudson-Civetta, 1996). The use of a pathway that outlines the entire treatment episode from prehospital care to posthospital services can increase consumers' confidence in the health care system while increasing cost-efficiency and quality outcomes. This is because both the care providers are more organized, and, when a copy of the clinical pathway is given to the patient, the daily expectations are clearly outlined (Mosher et al., 1992). This is expected to enhance patient satisfaction as the patient and family become involved consumers of care.

The goal of the clinical pathway is to outline a plan of care that describes the important elements of care from the time of admission, or before, to discharge, using specific time frames. It differs from the traditional focus on physician and nursing orders, which tend more toward a day-by-day focus, with terminal objectives not clearly explicated. The pathway provides a way for nurses and other health care providers to coordinate care and collaborate with the total health care team (Del Togno-Armanasco, 1995). The emphasis is on moving toward ensuring achievement of acceptable patient outcomes within an effective time frame with the appropriate use of resources (Mosher et al., 1992).

The Clinical Pathway as a Documentation Tool

Use of the Pathway as a Permanent Record

Spooner and Yockey (1996) suggest that the clinical pathway be made a permanent part of the patient record. When it is a permanent part of the record, it will be seen as an important information source and will be accorded more value. Many hospitals are struggling with a paper system for clinical pathways and are finding problems in obtaining compliance with their usage (Bultema et al., 1996; Spooner & Yockey, 1996). If the pathway were to become the primary mode of documentation, some of these problems might be alleviated.

An institution's documentation tools must support caregivers as they are asked to work more efficiently, decrease duplication, and increase quality of care. When a clinical pathway system is introduced, it must not be viewed as another piece of paper on which to chart. Charting requirements already demand too much of caregivers' precious time. If the clinical pathway is to be accepted by care providers as a documentation tool, it must replace the forms previously required. When it is used in this manner, less time will be spent in charting lengthy outcomes notes, leaving more time for direct patient care (Forkner, 1996).

Pathway Automation: Advantages for Nursing

Nurses have traditionally been the coordinators of patient care. When care was not given, or not documented by other disciplines, the nurse often assumed the responsibility to follow up with other providers to verify that the care was given. With automated clinical pathways, the role of the nurse is made easier. The accountability for assessment, interventions, and monitoring required of each discipline is explicit on the pathway. As each discipline provides care, this is documented on the computer record. Thus, the nurse no longer must be responsible for following up with other health care providers to make sure ordered treatments have been completed. For example, the physical therapist will document on the automated record that a patient who had a total hip repair was ambulated twice on Day 2. The nurse does not need to call a pharmacy to ensure that the patient has been taught how to use a metered dose inhaler before discharge because this teaching is documented on the computer record. The nurse no longer wonders if the diabetic educator has contacted the patient and what content was covered in the teaching session. With an automated record, the nurse can quickly see that each intervention has been provided as listed on the clinical pathway, and the outcome of the care is described.

Another goal of pathway automation is to streamline documentation requirements for care providers. When data is entered electronically into a computer, especially when it is in close proximity to the patient, care provider time is minimized. This allows practitioners more time for direct patient care because less time is spent on traditional documentation and communication (Kirton et al., 1996). In the current era of scarcity of health care resources, any effort to minimize non-patient-care activities for care providers is welcomed.

Implementation of an Automated Clinical Pathway at Flagstaff Medical Center

Flagstaff Medical Center (FMC), serving rural Northern Arizona, has attempted to reduce care provider documentation time by instituting a computerized charting system that uses the clinical pathway as both a guide for care and as a documentation tool. In the spring of 1996, the clinical pathways developed at FMC were automated on the Clinical Information System (CIS). This system is used to input, display, and report patient information. Computers are located at nearly every bedside as well as in nursing stations and ancillary provider departments. This close proximity of the computer to the place where patient care is provided facilitates data input at the time an assessment is made or the intervention is completed.

At FMC, the pathway has become an interdisciplinary care plan. Each discipline uses the clinical pathway to document the plan of care, individualize the plan of care, and set mutual outcome goals. Disciplines that document information on the pathway include nursing, physical therapy, pharmacy, dietary, case management, speech therapy, occupational therapy, home health, diabetic educators, and social work. Physician use of the pathway varies. Some use it as a reference; others for determining progress toward desired outcomes. This practice has enhanced communication between caregivers, and quality of care has increased as the mutual goals for the patient are shared.

At FMC, the assessments, interventions, education, discharge planning, and outcomes that should occur for a particular diagnosis are all included on the pathway. It also incorporates the interdisciplinary plan of care, patient education record, provider progress notes, and outcome documentation. Because the interventions and outcomes are preprinted on the pathway, the caregiver must only indicate when interventions are completed and whether the outcomes are met. This eliminates lengthy narrative notes and makes it more likely that the patient record contains the required documentation. Important elements of patient care that need to be documented are now present in the patient record, a situation not true prior to the use of the pathway as the documentation tool.

Interdisciplinary Clinical Pathway Development

To make the clinical pathway a documentation tool that all care providers will accept, it must be developed by an interdisciplinary team. To accomplish this, inclusion of all providers who will be involved in the care of the patient must be part of the development team. The varied disciplines must come together to identify the best practice for a particular disease state. Selection of criteria for inclusion in the pathway should start with collecting information about the specific illness, both from national databases and from local practice patterns. Historical trends from within the institution should also be examined. Review of interdisciplinary research concerning practice issues is also needed (Cole et al., 1996).

An example of a interdisciplinary team is that which developed a pathway for the care of a patient undergoing joint replacement. This pathway covered the period from the prehospital teaching program to discharge from either a rehabilitation program or home physical therapy services. The team that was brought together to develop this pathway included an orthopedic surgeon, a physiatrist, physical and occupational therapists, a pharmacist, an orthopedic nurse, a rehabilitation nurse, a presurgical nurse, and staff from the presurgical admitting area. The pathway that emerged from this teamwork reflected the best practices of each discipline involved in the care of the patient. When pathways are developed in this way, possible legal challenges that question the care a patient receives will be reduced.

There must also be an interdisciplinary commitment to the implementation, use, and ongoing evaluation and revision process of the clinical pathway. Locally created pathways should undergo an annual reassessment that includes a review of the literature to validate that the pathway reflects the most current practices. For the pathway to be effective and continue to provide liability protection, this annual review must include the physicians (Kennedy, 1996). When research advances knowledge in a particular patient management category, the new information must be incorporated into the pathway. Pathway content should also be automatically reevaluated when new clinical practice guidelines are issued by a medical professional group (Spath, 1996b).

Local Focus

The practices outlined in a pathway must reflect a local focus. This is particularly true in rural areas, where the depth of services available in an urban area is not present. Rural hospitals must decide which services can be provided locally and which services will need to be referred elsewhere, and the pathway must reflect these differences (Hicks & Bopp, 1996). The pathway then will reflect services locally available or through linkages with other providers. An important aspect of pathway use is to provide a coordinated plan for how the patient will access needed services, thus reducing the frustration that arises when services are fragmented. This is particularly important in rural areas, where patients often drive long distances to obtain health services. They need to be able to accomplish all of their testing and treatments at one time. Returning the next day to complete overlooked treatments is not an option. These principles can be shown in the following example, which uses the total hip replacement pathway developed at FMC.

The service area of FMC includes the local community as well as a large rural area stretching across central and eastern northern Arizona. There is an adequate number of physicians in the community to serve the needs of both Flagstaff residents and those in the surrounding communities, but these providers are not always easily accessible to patients in the rural areas. Rural elderly and poor are especially likely to have difficulty accessing health care providers because there is no public transportation infrastructure in the rural areas. One group in particular for which transportation is especially difficult is the Native American population on the Navajo Reservation. These people find it very difficult to travel to Flagstaff for needed medical services because of problems with both distance and limited economic resources.

When implementing the total hip pathway, these barriers to care had to be considered. The pathway includes a pre-op education class that prepares the patient for the recovery process by reviewing exercise and mobility techniques. Attendance at these classes may shorten the postoperative recovery period and possibly prevent complications. However, in northern Arizona, it is difficult for patients from rural areas to attend the pre-op class because of lack of transportation and the unaffordability of a motel room. To address the transportation issues, the surgeon's office staff works with the hospital to coordinate the needed services, preadmissions visit, and the pre-op education class on the same day to eliminate duplicate trips to Flagstaff for the patient. The case manager may set up a voucher system for patients to defray the expense of a motel room. The logistics of how a patient will be able to meet the treatments outlined on the pathway are as important to the pathway's development as the treatment plan itself.

Outcome-Focused Care

The simultaneous focus of managed care organizations on quality and cost effectiveness creates a challenging climate for health professionals. Payers for health care, led by large employers and insurance companies, are demanding clinical, financial, and satisfaction outcomes from providers. A philosophical shift is occurring, from a focus on episodes of care to the delivery of processes of care by teams of health care personnel (Campion & Rosenblatt, 1996). Hospital restructuring must address organizational system issues that facilitate control of the care delivery process and enhance quality. Staff at all levels of the organization must be involved in producing, supporting, and monitoring quality (Olivas, Del Togno-Armanasco, Erickson, & Harter, 1989). The quality management program needs to be a coordinated effort in which representatives from all disciplines that provide care to a patient work collaboratively to measure the outcomes of that care. This collaborative effort is encouraged in the 1995 Joint Commission of Accreditation of Health Care Organizations (JCAHO) standards, which seek greater collaboration and less focus on department-specific outcome indicators (Campion & Rosenblatt, 1996). Outcome measures based on standards found on the clinical pathways provide the means for analyzing care delivery from several perspectives, including those of the patient, family, and payers (Gelinas & Manthey, 1995).

At FMC, the automated pathway has specific areas for outcome documentation, variance documentation, and discharge criteria. Six to eight outcome measures are identified as quality indicators for each pathway and are measured on a monthly basis, using aggregate data. These data are reported on a quarterly basis to the Clinical Pathways Committee, Quality Council, medical staff committees, and unit-based council meetings. In this way, the clinical pathway is an integral part of the quality management program. Additional indicators are being developed to identify length of stay and cost issues associated with each pathway as measures of resource utilization.

The variance analysis process is used to identify problems at the patient level at an early stage. A variance occurs when a patient does not meet a predetermined expected outcome on the pathway. Variances can be viewed as negative or positive. A negative variance may delay care and result in a poor patient outcome. A positive variance may demonstrate an improved patient outcome and contribute to early discharge. The health care provider will attempt to address a negative variance at the time of the event. If not resolved, the variance will be analyzed by the pathway team as part of the quality management program. When negative variances persist, aggregate data are used to alert physicians, unit directors, and quality managers to possible problems in care so that a solution can be found before the problem becomes a major issue.

Example of an Automated Clinical Pathway

To illustrate how the computerized charting system uses a clinical pathway, the following figures are included. Figure 9.1 is a paper copy of the clinical pathway for a patient undergoing a total hip replacement. On it are identified those activities expected to happen, starting with preadmission and finishing with postdischarge follow-up. Figure 9.2 is an example of an automated screen that has been printed from the CIS and identifies activities performed on the immediate post-op day. Key interventions are followed by a choice list. From this list, the nurse selects the choice that indicates the intervention that is pertinent to the individual patient. In this example, the nurse chose "IV

Total Hip Clinical Pathway

***This pathway is a general guideline only, care is individualized and revised based upon the unique needs of the patient.**

Day	Pre-Admission Day	Day of Surgery	Post-Op Day 1	Post-Op Day 2	Post-Op Day 3	Post-Op Day 4	Follow-Up
Diet	Instruct on NPO status prior to surgery.	NPO pre-op. Diet as tolerated post-op.	Diet as tolerated. Diet consult if indicated.	Diet as tolerated.	Diet as tolerated.	Diet as tolerated.	NA
Consults	Medicine Consult. Surgeon's office will schedule patient to attend Joint Replacement Class.	RN will notify Soc. Worker of consult. Notify PT of consult.	PT consult completed. Soc. Ser. consult completed. Notify OT, Physiatry of consult.	OT consult. Physiatry consult.	NA	NA	NA
Tests	CBC, EKG, CXR, UA, Type & Cross, Pre-Albumin, PT, PTT, Chem 7. Draw fresh clot.	AP & Lat of pelvis of operative side.	Hemogram.	Hemogram.	Hemogram\ venous ultrasound.	NA	NA
Activity	As tolerated.	Bedrest with hip precautions.	Exercises, gait training, and precautions per PT.	PT BID for exercises-minimal assist.	PT BID for assisted ambulation.	Ambulatory.	NA
Medications	As per physician. Discuss pain scale and importance of pain control. Give "Pain Control After Surgery" guide to patient.	IV or hep lock until PO intake 500cc. Antibiotics X 48 hrs post-op. Pain meds and anti-emetics. Enoxaparin Q 12 hrs.	Antibiotics as ordered. LOC and vitamins. Pain meds as ordered. Enoxaparin Q 12 hrs.	LOC, vitamins. Pain meds as ordered. D\C IV. Enoxaparin Q 12 hrs.	LOC, vitamins, pain meds. Cont Enoxaparin if U\S pos for DVT.	LOC, vitamins. Pain meds as ordered.	NA
Nursing Care	Referrals to notify SNF\Rehab of possible admissions.	Routine po vital signs. Neuro-vasc checks to lower ext q 2 hrs. Blood replacement as ordered. Reinforce dressing prn. O2 to maintain sats 90%. IS q 1 hr W/A. Foley or straight cath q 6 hrs prn urinary retention. SCDS bilaterally.	Neuro-vasc checks. SCDS bilaterally. O2 to maintain sats 90%. IS q 1 hr W\A. Hemovac drain care. Blood replacement as ordered.	D\C hemovac. Wound care. SCDS. Incentive spirometer. O2 to maintain sats 90%. D\C foley. Blood replacement as ordered.	Wound care.	Wound care.	F\U phone call by One-Call RN.
Discharge Planning	Assess support systems and home environment.	Assess discharge planning needs.	Discharge plan complete. Notify Home Health if indicated.	Finalize SNF\ Rehab transfer if indicated.	SNF\Rehab transfer if appropriate.	Discharge to home if appropriate.	NA
Teaching	Give Total Hip Education packet and copy of patient-friendly pathway. Complete consent for surgery, anesthesia questionnaire, and pre-op checklist. Explain anatomy and function of surgical area.	Reinforce coughing and deep breathing. Instruct on use of PCA pump, and document pain level on vital signs screen.	Instruct on S\S of complications and when to call MD. Instruct on wound care. Instruct on exercises, ambulation\transfer techniques, and use of equipment.	Reinforce previous teaching.	Hip precautions, toilet transfer, adaptive devices, & ADL's. If not independent, care giver will demonstrate ability to assist pt.	Rein force previous teaching. Instruct on F/U appt with MD. Complete discharge instruction sheet.	NA

Figure 9.1 Clinical Pathway: Total Hip

Note Time: N/A
Topic:
Mode: Entry

Return to Clinical Pathway list by exiting this document, "Control F6", "new note", request the Total Hip Reference Pathway, and "print". This printed copy is to be placed with the Kardex and used as a reference in change of shift report. This is a worksheet which the nurses can make notes on, highlight interventions that have been completed, and discard once the patient is discharged.

ADMISSION NOTE	Received into 314 post-op at 1400. Wife at bedside. States pain level is a "3".			
		Intervention status	Notes	Var
Diagnostic Studies	AP & LAT pelvis of operative side in PACU.			☐
Nutrition	Regular diet as tolerated. with high iron/fiber		☐	
Consults	RN to notify Social Worker of consult (ext. 12220).			
	Notify Physical Therapy of consult (place order using order entry system)		☐	☐
Activity	Bedrest, Hip precautions, Keep legs abducted, Knee immobilizer		☐	☐
Medication	IV TKO or heplock until PO intake > 500 cc.	IV infusing as ordered		
	Antibiotics X 48 hrs Post-Op.	Not ordered		
	Enoxaparin 30 mg SQ Q 12 hr.	Ordered		
	Pain medication as ordered.	Pain med IV push		
	Document pain level (1-10), pre and post pain medication administration, on vital signs flowsheet.			
	Anti-emetics as ordered.	Anti-emetic IV	☐	x
Variance	health care provider	Physician did not order an antibiotic.		
Education	Assure Total Hip Education Packet is at bedside.	Packet at bedside	☐	☐
Interventions	* Routine Post-OP Vitals: Q15 min X 4, Q 30min X 4, Qhr X 4, * Q4 hrs X 48 hrs. * Neurovascular checks to lower ext Q 2 hr (document on * assessment flowsheet) * Reinforce dressing PRN * Homovac drain compressed, Empty Q8 hrs and PNR * O2 PRN to keep sats > 90% * Incentive spirometer Q 1 hr while awake * Foley cath or straight cath Q6 hrs PRN urinary retention			
	Administer blood replacement per hospital policy.	not ordered		
	DVT prophylaxis ordered:	TED hose Bilaterally	☐	☐
Outcome	* At 6 hours post-op, after intervention for pain, pain level will be documented on VS screen.	Outcomes met - pain level 4 or less		☐

Interdisciplinary Progress/Outcome Note for Day of Surgery Post-Op

Document outcome note addressing pain every 24 hours.

Progress/Outcome Evaluation

01

Figure 9.2 Automated Screen—Post-Op Day 1: Total Hip Pathway

infusing as ordered" from the choice list. However, antibiotics were not ordered as outlined on the pathway, resulting in a health care provider variance, which was documented. Also listed on this screen is an educational intervention and other key interventions required for the care of this patient. Also listed is an expected outcome related to pain management. The nurse indicated that this outcome was met; the patient's pain level was at 4 or less on a scale of 10.

Figure 9.3 is an example of an automated screen that shows a portion of the post-op Day 3. Physical therapy interventions are outlined, followed by physical therapy documentation. All interventions were completed except for education in tub transfers. This intervention was not appropriate for this patient, and a patient-related variance was documented.

This example of a computerized patient record, using the clinical pathway as the guide to care provision, demonstrates how a multidisciplinary record of care can be generated. Use of a record such as this provides all care providers with an up-to-the-minute report of the patient's progress. Because each aspect of care is included and must be addressed, the record of care for the patient will not be ambiguous. If, at a later date, there is a question about the care received, a legible, complete record is available. Such documentation should decrease the likelihood of legal problems for the providers if a malpractice issue were to arise.

Legal Implications

As the clinical pathway begins to serve not only as a quality management tool but also as a documentation tool that is a permanent part of the patient record, liability concerns have been raised. Health professionals worry that a clinical pathway will be used as evidence in a court of law. Plaintiffs' attorneys are very aware of the existence of clinical pathways. Some physicians at FMC question the practice of outlining patient care goals and including them in the chart for fear that such documentation will later be used against them in a court of law. Because the pathway is a generic plan of care for patients with a specific diagnosis, the plan may not be appropriate for all patients. The question to consider is if the physician decides not to follow the plan, are there potential legal considerations? This concern is widespread across the country (Cole et al., 1996).

Note Time: N/A
Topic:
Mode: Entry

Date | Discipline | Problem | Progress/Outcome Evaluation
#1
Physician Progress Notes

POST-OP DAY THREE Date 6/18/98 Intervention Status Notes Var

Diagnostic Studies — Hemogram, Venous ultrasound

Nutrition — Regular diet as tolerated with high iron/fiber

Activity

Contact SW to make Home Health referral if indicated and not being transferred to SNF/Rehab — 3.Home Health referral made

TO BE COMPLETED BY PT/OT

Therapeutic exercise with stand-by assist > contact guard assist. — #1 Completed

Supine to sit, minimal contact guard assist. Sit to stand contact guard assist. — #1 Completed

Gait 50 ft w/ stand-by assist. Indicate if patient reaches goal of 75 ft. — #1 Completed

Demonstrate hip precautions without verbal cues. — #1 Completed

Complies with weight bearing status — #1 Completed

Education in toilet transfers — #1 meets goals/outcomes

Educate in tub transfer — #1 not completed (see variance)

Educate in adaptive devices — #1 meets goals/outcomes

Educate in dressing, hygiene, grooming — #1 meets goals/outcomes

Total time of PT visit #1 45 min Therapist/Tech #1 B. Bonner X

Nursing-assisted activities: X

#1 at 12:00, patient assisted up to chair by nursing for lunch. Patient transferred with contact guard assist while observing hip precautions.

Variance patient-related — Patient not instructed in tub transfer, as is obese and transfer to tub is hazardous. Patient will be showering when returning to home.

Medication
- MVI w/ minerals PO daily
- FeSO4 1 PO BID
- LOC
- Pain medication as ordered

Figure 9.3 Automated Screen—Post-Op Day 3: Total Hip Pathway

SOURCE: Copyright © 1998 Flagstaff Medical Center. Used by permission.

Negligence is a general term referring to a deviation from a standard of care that a reasonable person would use in a particular set of circumstances. Malpractice is a more specific type of negligence. It is a deviation from a professional standard of care. To prove that malpractice or negligence has occurred, four elements must be established: duty, breach of duty, causation, and damages (Fiesta, 1993). Clinical pathways focus on the breach-of-duty element that occurs when a standard of care has not been met. If a caregiver does not meet the standard of care because he or she did not follow the clinical pathway, this could be evidence of malpractice.

However, having a clinical pathway in place and available as a quick reference, the provider has the opportunity to document the reason for a deviation from the pathway at the time of the care decision. Such documentation should strengthen, rather than weaken, the provider's position (Cole et al., 1996). A jury could see that the standards outlined on the pathway were considered and reasons for not following these standards were explained through variance analysis. Even if the outcome does not turn out as expected, the rationale for the choices made can be identified (Kennedy, 1996). However, if the care is consistent with the pathway and a negative situation occurs, attorneys may be deterred from bringing suit altogether (Courlas, 1996). Many who support clinical pathways believe they will decrease the practice of defensive medicine by providing liability protection (Courlas, 1996).

Standard of Care

Clinical pathways are another source, like expert witnesses, for attorneys and judges to use to establish standards of care (Courlas, 1996). Some physicians view this as a reason not to have the clinical pathway in the patient record. However, if a clinical pathway is not used, other means of outlining the standard of care will be introduced in court. The lack of a locally created clinical pathway allows the plaintiff's attorney to choose from many hundreds of pathways developed across the country to introduce as evidence. In effect, he or she could choose a pathway that best reinforces the plaintiff's case (Kennedy, 1996). According to Spath (1996a), with or without pathways, clinicians are expected to meet the community standard of care or justify their reason for varying from that standard. All clinicians need to understand the importance of documenting deviations from professional standards of care to prevent malpractice litigation.

Locally Created Pathways

Traditionally, in malpractice, the practitioner is held to the standard of care of a professional practicing in the same geographical area (Fiesta, 1993). The hospital and its employees must exercise toward the patient that degree of skill, care, and diligence used by hospitals generally in the community where the hospital in question is located or in similar communities. A clinical pathway can be considered the community standard of care because it was created and approved by the local care providers and physicians. However, the law is now moving toward a national standard, which would hold a practitioner from any area in the country to a nationally established standard of care. The community cannot set a standard that is below the nationally accepted standard (Fiesta, 1993).

For a rural community, the pathway must reflect the national standard of care and outline how that standard can be accomplished within the limitations of a rural environment. It may not be possible to achieve the same level of testing or the time standards for initiating treatment found in an urban environment. For example, it is often not possible to have emergency medical services available to a rural population in a timely manner to manage a person with a possible myocardial infarction, as is found in the urban area. However, if a service cannot be provided locally in a rural area, a mechanism must be in place to ensure that the services are available through linkages with other health care providers (Hicks & Bopp, 1996).

Deviation From the Standard of Care

The pathway should be viewed as a guideline for care. It not a standard of care that should be followed for every patient. Individualization of the pathway is encouraged and must occur to adjust to the unique needs of the patient. To lessen the risk of liability claims, hospitals should print a disclaimer on each pathway. At FMC, the following disclaimer, as recommended by Spath (1996b), is printed in the pathway policies.

> These clinical guidelines are designed to assist clinicians by providing an analytical framework for the evaluation and treatment of patients and are not intended either to replace a clinician's judgment or to establish a protocol for all patients with a particular condition. (p. 126)

Whether the law is dealing with a physician or a nurse, the issue of standard of care and duty should be to consider how a reasonable professional would have acted in a similar situation. If individual circumstances indicate deviation from the standard, the reasons should be documented (Hall, 1996). Clear documentation of the variance in the chart is more credible than an undocumented verbal explanation during a trial (Forkner, 1996). Variance explanations on a clinical pathway can be a powerful mechanism to prevent malpractice litigation (Forkner, 1996).

Legal and Accurate Record

The need for clear and complete documentation is enforced in licensure statutes and regulations, as well as by malpractice law. The standard for documentation is that there must be an accurate record of the patient's condition and care. Documentation must be objective, clear, accurate, and complete. Computerized documentation is accepted as legal if it meets the standard of an accurate record of condition and care (Hall, 1996). It has also been by approved by the JCAHO as an acceptable charting format for nursing documentation (Mosher et al., 1992).

Malpractice cases often hinge on documentation. If the patient record is not complete because the caregiver failed to document assessments or interventions, the lack of documentation may create a presumption that the care was not given. Omissions in charting are frequent problems from the malpractice defense standpoint. Frequently, an omission in the patient record leads to an allegation that the care provider breached the standards of care. Good documentation is considered good nursing practice. Nurses who are expert witnesses for the patient-plaintiff may use poorly kept nurses' notes as a support for a conclusion that the patient was poorly monitored by the nursing staff (Hall, 1996). A jury may correlate a sloppy, disorganized record with sloppy, disorganized care.

The use of the clinical pathway as a documentation tool can overcome many of the problems found in care provider charting. Because documentation using a clinical pathway promotes charting by exception, there is less chance of not including a vital piece of information. The interventions are outlined on the pathway, and the outcome note may be written, "care provided as per clinical pathway." This can reduce the chance of documentation errors. Another positive reason for using the clinical pathway as a documentation tool is that the clinical pathway outlines the expected interventions in a simple format that is easy for a jury to follow (Forkner, 1996). When such clarity can be provided, one's practice may be easier to defend in a malpractice case.

Legal Considerations for Use of Computer Documentation System

Use of a computerized charting system brings with it a number of legal issues that must be addressed. Patient confidentiality is a prime issue to consider. It is the responsibility of each clinical information system user to guarantee the privacy of the patient's medical record. All chart information is confidential and must only be accessed by persons with a security access password.

Because at FMC the computer terminals are located in each patient room, special precautions are needed to provide the necessary security for them. If a terminal will be unattended, the user must manually lock the screen before leaving the room. Another safeguard is that if the screen has not been used for five minutes, it will become blank, and a password will be required to access the system.

Written consent of the patient or his legally qualified representative is required for the release of medical information to persons not otherwise authorized to receive information. All hard copies of material generated from any computer system must be regarded with the same level of confidentiality as on-line information. Printed material cannot be left unattended in areas where it can be accessed by unauthorized individuals. Nonpermanent printouts of confidential information must be destroyed according to hospital policy.

Appropriate access to computer system information is defined as that which is necessary for the employee to perform job duties. Access is restricted to individuals who have need, reason, and permission to access such information. Caregivers who are permitted to access the computer system information are required to sign a computer system confidentiality agreement. Any access to computer system information beyond the scope of a caregiver's responsibilities is considered a security violation and may result in disciplinary action. Leaving a computer logged in and unattended for any period of time that might allow an unauthorized person to gain access is not permissible.

Each caregiver uses an electronic signature that identifies that person whenever he or she enters the chart. This is done by providing each person with a unique password. This password can be used to access the system and enter or edit data. The electronic signature, which consists of the full last name, full first name, title, and initials, will be attached to data stored when the password is used. The systems manager is able to review information entered or edited on a patient's record and can identify the responsible caregiver. Thus, when a patient record is used for any review purpose, the caregiver responsible for each aspect of care can be readily identified.

The electronic record can be edited by the caregiver to correct information or spelling prior to storing information. Information can also be corrected after storage. If a change is needed to correct information on the record, data fields can be edited by anyone with password access. The automated record will then display both the altered and unaltered forms. All entries in the automated record have a time, date, and name stamp associated with them. Late entries will be placed in chronological order, and the date and time of the late entry will be shown.

The use of a computerized charting system allows for use by a number of disciplines. Because the chart is available at every computer terminal, each care provider who needs access to it can do so in a timely manner. There is no waiting for someone else to finish using the chart or to spend time hunting for it. Another advantage of this type of charting is that the various disciplines do their charting in the same section of the chart. A natural outcome of this is increased interdisciplinary accountability, communication, and collaboration. It provides a system of checks and balances that can cut down on workload, promote quality care, and, ultimately, save the patient time and money (Kirton et al., 1996). This system of charting is a highly acceptable alternative to the usual method of segregated documentation of observations and treatment by each discipline. Integrated charting is also preferable for legal reasons, because the courts presume that all disciplines read each others' notes, and any procedure that will make it easier for that process to occur is commendable (Fiesta, 1983).

Conclusions

Consumer satisfaction hinges on an organization's ability to deliver quality care in an organized, cost-effective, and compassionate manner (Bultema et al., 1996). Patient satisfaction surveys (Murphy, 1995) indicate that patients want their health care system to be less fragmented and more collaborative and continuous in its service. The typical malpractice suit centers around an "unsatisfied customer," so any system that can increase communication and consistency in patient care is to be commended.

Clinical pathways, in one form or another, are increasingly becoming a part of patient care delivery systems. The emergence of the computer as the primary vehicle for managing information and disseminating it is also part of our new reality: It is necessary to inform and connect people in all kinds of environments. As clinical pathways and computers merge, effective automated plans of care that can also serve as documentation tools will benefit both the caregiver and the patient and decrease the risk of liability. This combination may well be an important means to prevent malpractice litigation.

Effective information management systems are increasingly becoming a part of the managed health care environment. These systems can increase efficiency in documentation so providers will have more time for direct patient interaction. They can also be used for quality management tracking, through the use of variance analysis, so problems within the system can be detected early and corrections can be made. Data that support claims that the clients enrolled in a particular health care organization to achieve positive health outcomes will enhance that organization's reputation—a vital component to the success of the organization.

References

Bultema, J. K., Mailliard, L., Getzfrid, M. K., Lerner, R. D., & Colone, M. (1996). Geriatric patients with depression: Improving outcomes using a multidisciplinary clinical path model. *Journal of Nursing Administration, 26*, 31-38.

Cole, L., Lasker-Hertz, S., Grady, G., Clark, M., & Houston, S. (1996). Structured care methodologies: Tools for standardization and outcomes measurement. *Nursing Case Management, 1*(4), 160-172.

Campion, F. X., & Rosenblatt, M. S. (1996). Quality assurance and medical outcomes in the era of cost containment. *Surgical Clinics of North America, 76*, 139-159.

Courlas, S. D. (1996). Clinical practice guidelines coming on strong! Managed care requires the development of systems. *Healthcare Perspectives, 5*, 1-7.

Del Togno-Armanasco, V. (1995). Let's trash the care plan! *Nursing Management, 26*, 54.

Fiesta, J. (1983). *The law and liability: Guide for nurses*. New York: Wiley.

Forkner, J. (1996). Clinical pathways, benefits and liabilities. *Nursing Management, 26*, 35-37.

Gelinas, L. S., & Manthey, M. (1995). Improving patient outcomes through system change: A focus on the changing roles of healthcare organization executives. *Journal of Nursing Administration, 25*, 55-58.

Hall, J. K. (1996). *Nursing ethics and law*. Philadelphia: W. B. Saunders.

Hicks, L. L., & Bopp, K. D. (1996). Integrated pathways for managing rural health services. *Health Care Management Review, 21*, 65-72.

Kirton, O. C., Civetta, J. M., & Hudson-Civetta, J. (1996). Cost effectiveness in the intensive care unit. *Surgical Clinics of North America, 76*, 175-200.

Kennedy, E. K. (1996). Critical pathways and practice guidelines can be a liability nightmare. *Assertive Utilization Management Report, 6*, 1-3.

Mosher, C., Cronk, P., Kidd, A., McCormick, P., Stockton, S., & Sulla, C. (1992). Upgrading practice with critical pathways. *American Journal of Nursing, 92*, 41-44.

Murphy, L. (1995). Mercy Healthcare's CARE 2000: An evolution in progress. *Nursing Administration Quarterly, 20*, 47-48.

Olivas, G. S., Del Togno-Armanasco, V., Erickson, J. R., & Harter, S. (1989). Case management: A bottom-line care delivery model. *Journal of Nursing Administration, 19*, 16-20.

Spath, P. (1996a). Clinical pathways: No smoking gun for malpractice cases. *Hospital Peer Review, 21*(8), 113-115.

Spath, P. (1996b). Lessen your path-related liability concerns. *Hospital Peer Review, 21*(9), 125-127.

Spooner, S. H., & Yockey, P. S. (1996). Assessing clinical pathway effectiveness: A model for evaluation. *Nursing Case Management, 1*, 188-198.

Chapter

10

Clinical Pathway Outcome Research

Pamela Keberlein

Accurate knowledge is the basis of correct opinion.
C. Simmons (Catrevas, Edwards, & Browns, 1963)

Clinical pathways (also called critical pathways) have emerged as a tool for nursing to use to better track patients' progress through an acute hospital stay. It is expected that increased efficiency and lowered costs will result from this (Horne, 1996). At the same time, managed care organizations have mandated that quality health care be provided more efficiently. Services and resources must be managed so that clinical benefits are maximized while costs are minimized (Boles & Fleming, 1996). However, little research has been done to examine the effects of clinical pathway usage on costs and quality outcomes. Without such research, the effect of clinical pathways on patient outcomes remains in the realm of opinion rather than fact.

Clinical pathways have been extolled as one way to track the delivery of patient care so that resource utilization will be maximized and the quality of the care can be evaluated (Kegal, 1996). However, this is a very new area of research and new methods to study these issues are just beginning to be developed. The majority of studies that have looked at the effect of the use of clinical pathways on patient outcomes have focused on cost issues and not on quality outcomes. Pearson, Goulart-Fisher, and Lee (1995) suggest there are significant gaps in knowledge between the projected effect of pathways on reduced costs and improved quality of care. Thus, there is a great need to thoroughly examine the effects of the use of clinical pathways on patient outcomes and quality of care.

Another demand of the managed care environment is that nurses demonstrate greater efficiency, productivity, and cost efficiency (Girouard, 1996). Methods to measure outcomes of care using tools such as clinical pathways are one way to demonstrate the effect of nursing interventions on patient outcomes. Another way is to look at resource utilization as a measure to demonstrate cost savings.

This chapter will present a study designed to measure the effects of the introduction of clinical pathways into an acute-care hospital setting on both resource utilization and quality outcome measures. The clinical pathways were developed by a multidisciplinary team under the direction of an advanced practice nurse. Another advanced practice nurse was responsible for directing the care of patients using the clinical pathways. Resource utilization will be examined by looking at length-of-stay (LOS) issues and cost for the hospitalization. The changes in resource utilization must consider both people and products. Quality of care provided will be examined by comparing patient outcomes achieved with preselected outcomes on the clinical pathway. In this chapter, these areas will be explored to find answers to the pressing questions of the managed care health environment.

Examples of Outcome Studies

The literature is permeated with reports describing the effects of the use of clinical pathways. It is suggested that clinical pathways improve collaboration among departments (Bigos Graybeal, Gheen, & McKenna, 1993), enhance patient and staff satisfaction (Goode, 1995), improve efficiency and promote an ideal plan of care (Spath, 1995), and provide a forum for the merging of clinical and financial knowledge to improve the process of care (Shikiar & Warner, 1994; Wall, Joseph, & MacGrath, 1993). However, the number of scientific studies that examine the effects of clinical pathways on patient outcomes is fairly limited.

DeWoody and Price (1994) describe the development of a clinical pathway for use with trauma patients. They examined changes in LOS following introduction of the pathway and found a decrease of 0.81 days. Even this small amount of change was found to make a significant impact on hospital revenues. Another study (Wentworth & Atkinson, 1996) looked at the effect of the implementation of a clinical pathway on 414 Medicare stroke patients. A decrease in acute-care LOS of 2.4 days was found when using the pathway. The patients were moved more rapidly into a rehabilitation situation than had occurred prior to the use of the pathway (Wentworth & Atkinson, 1996). Decreases in both LOS and hospital costs were found in a study of 47 patients undergoing carotid endarterectomy following introduction of a clinical pathway (Collier et al., 1995). Schoenenberger, Pearson, Goldhaber, and Lee (1996) investigated the use of a clinical pathway for patients with deep vein thrombosis. In their study of 92 patients, the pathway that promoted the use of timely anticoagulation revealed improved patient outcomes, both in decreased LOS and improved patient function.

Kowal and Delaney (1996) examined outcomes for patients undergoing mastectomy before and after the initiation of a clinical pathway. They used a convenience sample of 31 patients prior to use of the pathway and 31 patients after implementation of the pathway. Data collected in this study were hospital charges and LOS. Variances from the expected activities stated on the pathway were also examined. A significant decrease in both LOS and hospital charges was found following initiation of the pathway.

Many of these studies suggest that the use of clinical pathways improves quality of care and reduces resource utilization, but further study is needed. Pearson et al. (1995) state, "The gaps in our knowledge about critical pathways are excessive" (p. 941). Much of the literature describing outcomes achieved by use of clinical pathways is anecdotal. Additional research is needed to demonstrate the effects of use of clinical pathways on both quality of care and resource utilization.

Research Study

This study was conducted in a small, 108-bed community hospital in rural Arizona. Clinical pathways were introduced in this facility in 1996 as a means to manage patient care in an efficient manner and, at the same time, provide quality care. It was hoped that through their use, inefficient system practices could be reduced and overuse of resources would be prevented. This study was designed to investigate whether these expectations could be validated.

The pathways chosen for use in this study were those developed for use with patients with either congestive heart failure (CHF) or total hip replacement (THR). These two diagnoses were chosen because patients undergoing a THR represent an area of significant loss for the hospital. These patients have tended to have a relatively long length of stay in which the hospital charges exceeded the DRG reimbursement. In 1996, the mean charge for patients having a total hip replacement was $20,371; the Medicare reimbursement figure was $8,336. Patients with CHF have a pattern of frequent readmission, often within 15 days of discharge (Reiley & Howard, 1995).

Research Questions

In this study, several research questions were asked that related to the issues of resource utilization and quality outcomes. The effect of the use of a clinical pathway on hospital charges through looking at resource utilization prior to and after implementation of the pathway was a major portion of the study. The effect of the use of clinical pathways on achieving predetermined patient outcomes was also studied. An additional question, related to identification of variances from pathway guidelines, was also proposed; however, no usable data was found when looking at documentation variances. Limited documentation was present relating to variance analysis. This was attributed to the newness of the concept of variance for most of the staff. This is an area that requires considerably more education for all of the staff before consistency in documentation will be found.

Study Design

The study consisted of retrospective chart review of patients admitted with the two diagnoses, 6 months prior to the initiation of the clinical pathway and for a 6-month period following introduction of the pathway. The time period used provided for a 6-month period for the hospital staff to learn to use the pathways before the postpathway portion of the study was initiated. All patients admitted with either of the diagnoses were included in the study. The CHF sample comprised 57 patients for the prepathway group and 54 for the postpathway group. The THR sample consisted of 25 patients in the prepathway group and 19 patients in the postpathway group. The data collected included

Resource utilization
- Hospital charges from each department providing services
- Total hospital charges
- Length of stay
- Readmission data

Patient outcomes
- Hospital day discharge planning was begun
- Functional status
- Reasons for delay if discharge did not occur on scheduled day
- Patient education provided
- THR—day physical therapy treatment initiated
- CHF—daily weights obtained

Study Results: Congestive Heart Failure Group

All hospital charts for patients admitted with the diagnosis of congestive heart failure during the study periods were audited retrospectively by the researcher. Data reflecting both resource utilization and quality outcomes measures were collected and analyzed. The prepathway group consisted of 57 patients with a mean age of 72.9 years (*SD* = 10.19). The postpathway group included 54 patients with a mean age of 75.1 years (*SD* = 11.08). The results of this data analaysis are shown in Table 10.1.

Resource utilization

The mean length of stay for patients admitted with CHF prior to the introduction of the clinical pathway was 3.86 days; postpathway this time was reduced to 3.35 days. This decrease was determined not to be statistically significant even though it does indicate a trend in the desired direction in terms of resource utilization. Five of the patients in the postpathway group were classified as requiring maximum assistance with activities of daily living, an event that is well known to extend a person's hospital stay (Reiley & Howard, 1995). No patients in the prepathway group were identified as requiring maximum assistance with activities of daily living. However, in reviewing the

TABLE 10.1 Comparison of Data: Congestive Heart Failure Group

	Prepathway	*Postpathway*
N	57	54
Mean age	72.9 years (*SD* = 10.19)	75.1 years (*SD* = 11.08)
Outcome: Resource utilization		
Length of stay	3.86 days	3.35 days
2 or more hospital readmissions within 6 months of discharge	38.7% (22)[a]	16.8% (9)
Cost of care	$8,257	$8,524
Cost of care adjusted for rate increase (1996 dollars)	$8,257	$8,098
Number of patients undergoing cardiac catheterization	19.3% (11)	11.0% (6)
Outcome: Quality care		
Documentation of patient education	12.3% (7)	70.4% (38)
Documentation of daily weight	33.3% (19)	50.0% (27)
Demonstrated weight decrease	21.1% (12)	35.2% (19)
Documentation of discharge plan	24.0% (14)	57.9% (33)
Stay longer than 3 days	43.9% (25)	35.2% (19)

a. Numbers in parentheses represent actual number of patients.

data without these five patients included in the postpathway group, there was still no significant differnce in LOS between the two groups. Thus, it must be concluded that the introduction of the pathway had no effect on patient LOS.

A positive indication of the success of the use of the pathway was in the change in hospital readmission between the two groups. In the prepathway group, 38.7% (22 patients) had two or more admissions, and 11 of these had three or more admissions. In the postpathway group, only 16.8% (9 patients) had multiple admissions, and only 5 patients had more than three admissions during that time. This is a highly significant finding: Under a capitated payment system, a decrease in hospital admissions in a population with a chronic illness is a strategically important outcome.

Other indicators of resource utilization included the cost of care. This was looked at by each department of service that generated a patient charge. There was great variability in hospital charges between the two time periods. However, when that total patient charge is evaluated, the cost of the stay increased from $8,257 in the prepathway period to $8,524 in the postpathway period. However, an overall rate increase of 5% occurred between these two periods. When the 1997 rate is calculated at 1996 dollars, this cost comes to $8,098, a rate lower than that of the prepathway group. No statistical difference was found between these two rates. Another change found in resource utilization was a decrease in the number of patients in the postpathway group who underwent a cardiac catheterization procedure. In the prepathway group, 19.3% (11 patients) had this procedure done; in the postpathway group, only 11% (6 patients) had it done. This is an interesting trend that needs to be followed.

Quality Outcomes

Although the data for resource utilization was equivocal, the data related to quality outcomes demonstrates a positive effect of the pathways. In the area of documentation of patient education, only 12.3% (7 patients) of the prepathway group charts had patient education documented. The percentage for documentation of education in the postpathway group increased to 70.4% (338 patients), a significant increase. All patients now admitted with a diagnosis of CHF receive an education packet as well as a copy of the patient-friendly clinical path, which outlines specific areas for patient teaching as well as expected outcomes.

Another area of improvement is that of documentation of patient daily weights. In the prepathway group, only 33.3% (19 patients) of charts had weights recorded on a daily basis, and a mere 21.1% (12 patients) demonstrated a steady weight decline during their hospital stay. In the postpathway group, 50% (33 patients) of the charts had daily weights documented, and 35.2% (19 patients) showed a steady weight decline.

Discharge planning also improved dramatically. In the prepathway group, 24% (14 patients) had no discharge plan documented during their entire hospital stay. Although 57.9% (33 patients) had their plan begun on the first or second day, in the postpathway group, only 16.7% (9 patients) had no discharge plan and 79.2% (38 patients) had a discharge plan initiated by Day 2 of their hospital stay. Delay in discharge also showed some differences between the two groups. In the prepathway group, 43.9% (25 patients) had a hospital stay longer than 3 days; for 16 of these patients, no reason for the delay was documented. In the postpathway group, the percentage of patients whose stay was longer than 3 days was 35.2%; in all cases, the reason for the extended stay was documented. The reasons for delayed discharge included invasive procedures, use of vasoactive medications, unrelated medical problems, and, in one instance, failure to arrange for home health in a timely manner. Thus, only one of the delayed discharges was related to a system variance that could be corrected.

Study Results: Total Hip Replacement

The same strategies used with patients with congestive heart failure were used to study the effects of the introduction of clinical pathways on patients with total hip replacement. The sample used in this study consisted of 25 patients in the prepathway group and 19 patients in the postpathway group. The mean age of the patients in the prepathway group was 57.67 years (SD = 15.18) and in the postpathway group 66.52 years (SD = 12.69). These two groups were found to be significantly different in age ($p = .04$). The results of the analysis of data for the total hip replacement study are found in Table 10.2.

Resource Utilization

Resource utilization was compared between the patients undergoing a total hip replacement in the prepathway and the postpathway groups. The data reflecting mean length of stay actually increased in the postpathway group (5.21 days) over the prepathway group (4.24 days). Some of this difference may be related to the larger percentage of the postpathway group who were older than 60 years (74%); in the prepathway group, only 52% of the patients were 60 or older. Another significant difference between the groups was that the postpathway group included three patients with severe neurological conditions (stroke and Parkinson's disease).

Also, in the early stages of the THR pathway period, there was strong physician resistance to the use of the pathway, especially the pressure for early transfer to a skilled nursing facility (SNF) on the third postoperative day if it became clear that the patient would not be able to go directly home upon discharge. In the prepathway group, 43.9% (25 patients) had a hospital stay longer than 3 days; in the postpathway group, only 35.2% (19 patients) had hospital stays longer than 3 days. In the postpathway group, two patients experienced stays longer than 5 days because of delayed transfer to SNF. This has been identified as a problem area; as the result of these two incidents, discussions have been held to encourage all care providers to identify patients

TABLE 10.2 Comparison of Data: Total Hip Replacement Group

	Prepathway	*Postpathway*
N	25	19
Mean age[a]	57.67 years (*SD* = 15.18)	66.52 years (*SD* = 12.69)
Outcome: Resource utilization		
Length of stay	4.24 days	5.21 days
Hospital stay longer than 3 days	43.9% (25)	35.2% (19)
Cost of care	$20,371	$20,700
Cost of care adjusted for rate increase (1996 dollars)	$20,371	$19,665
Number of patients undergoing blood tranfusion and cell saver treatment	48% (12)	37% (7)
Outcome: Quality care		
Documentation of patient education	44% (11)	100% (19)
Documentation of physical therapy initiated on first post-operative day	88% (22)	94.7% (18)
Documentation of discharge plan	72% (18)	94.7% (18)
Readmission rate for deep vein thrombosis	8% (2)	5.3% (1)

a. $p = .04$.

who will need skilled nursing care early in the hospital stay and make plans to have them moved in a timely manner. Physician cooperation in this area is improving and LOS of these patients has decreased subsequent to this study.

The financial costs for the management of patients demonstrated an overall 3% decrease in total costs for the hospital when between the prepathway phase and postpathway phase. The mean cost of a hospital stay in the prepathway group was $20,371; the mean cost in the postpathway group was $20,700. When this figure is adjusted for 1996 dollars, it drops to $19,665. This difference was not significant. However, the Medicare reimbursement for this DRG in 1997 was $9,238; the mean total charge was $20,700, still indicating a substantial loss on each case. However, one change in a positive direction arose during the postpathway phases of the study. In the prepathway group, 48% (12) of the patients were treated with blood transfusions and a cell saver (the Brat 2, COBE) was used, a device used in surgery to capture the patient's own blood in a sterile container to be readministered to the patient. The use of these treatments did not appear to be correlated with postoperative hematocrits. In the postpathway group, only 37% (7) of patients were treated with both a cell saver and a transfusion of packed red cells. No patient with a hematocrit of more than 23 was given blood products. This change in practice resulted in a decrease in the total operating room costs.

Quality Outcomes

As with the CHF group, there was great improvement in patient outcomes and quality of care in the patients undergoing total hip replacement. In the prepathway group, 44% (11 patients) had education documented on the chart. In the postpathway group, all patients had at least partial completion of the patient education record, and 10 patients had all patient education documented. The pathway specifies that physical therapy activities should begin on the first postoperative day. This occurred in all but one of the postpathway patients, but in the prepathway group, three patients did not have their PT activities started until the second postoperative day.

In the prepathway group, 72% (18 patients) had a discharge plan documented prior to their discharge. In the postpathway group, all but one patient (94.7%) had a discharge plan documented. The discharge plan was initiated on Day 1 for 47.4% (9 patients) in the postpathway group; this occurred with only 1 (4%) of the prepathway group. The postdischarge readmission rate between the two groups was similar; 3 patients from each group were readmitted within 60 days. However, in the postpathway group, only one of these readmissions was for deep vein thrombosis, a possible complication of THR surgery. In the prepathway group, two of the readmissions were for deep vein thrombosis. A suggested possible reason for this difference could be related to the use of Enoxaparin, an anticoagulant drug listed on the pathway for suggested use.

Conclusions

Although there were small differences in resource utilization for the CHF and THR groups and some reduction in LOS for CHF patients after implementation of the clinical pathways, these changes were not found to be statistically significant. However, the decrease in readmission rates following implementation of the pathways is very positive. Also, the improvement found in the quality indicators is encouraging. The movement in reducing resource utilization and improving compliance with quality indicators suggests that implementation of clinical pathways may bring about desired institutional goals.

Because the timing of this study was so close to the time that the clinical pathways were implemented, this study may not be demonstrating the full potential that can be achieved with the use of the pathways. However, the design of the study can be used for subsequent monitoring. It may be possible that as all health care staff, including the physicians, become more comfortable with the use of clinical pathways, the positive movement to achieving organizational goals will be enhanced.

References

Bigos Graybeal, K., Gheen, M., & McKenna, B. (1993). Clinical pathway development: The Overlake model. *Nursing Management, 24*(4), 42-45.

Boles, K. E., & Fleming, S. T. (1996). Break even under capitation: Pure and simple? *Health Care Management Review, 21*(1), 38-47.

Catrevas, C. N., Edwards, J., & Browns, R. E. (Eds.). (1963). *The new dictionary of thought.* New York: Standard Book.

Collier, P. E., Friend, S. Z., Gentile, C., Ruckert, D., Vescio, L., & Collier, N. A. (1995). Carotid endarterectomy clinical pathway: An innovative approach. *American Journal of Medical Quality, 10*(1), 38-44.

DeWoody, S., & Price, J. (1994). A systems approach to multidimensional critical paths. *Nursing Management, 25*(11), 47-55.

Girouard, S. A. (1996). Evaluating advanced nursing practice. In A. B. Hamric, J. A. Spross, & C. M. Hanson (Eds.), *Advanced nursing practice: An integrative approach* (pp. 567-600). Philadelphia: Saunders.

Goode, C. J. (1995). Impact of a CareMap™ and case management on patient satisfaction and staff satisfaction, collaboration, and autonomy. *Nursing Economics, 13*(6), 337-348.

Horne, M. (1996). Involving physicians in clinical pathways: An example for perioperative knee arthroplasty. *Journal on Quality Improvement, 22*(2), 115-124.

Kegal, L. M. (1996). Case management, critical pathways, and myocardial infarction. *Critical Care Nurse, 16*(2), 97-112.

Kowal, N. S., & Delaney, M. (1996). The economics of a nurse-developed critical pathway. *Nursing Economics, 14*(3), 156-161.

Pearson, S. D., Goulart-Fisher, D., & Lee, T. H. (1995). Critical pathways as a strategy for improving care: Problems and potential. *Annals of Internal Medicine, 123*(12), 941-948.

Reiley, P., & Howard, E. (1995). Predicting hospital length of stay in elderly patients with congestive heart failure. *Nursing Economics, 13*(4), 210-216.

Schoenenberger, R. A., Pearson, S. D., Goldhaber, S. Z., & Lee, T. H. (1996). Variation in the management of deep vein thrombosis: Implications for the potential impact of a critical pathway. *American Journal of Medicine, 100,* 278-282.

Shikiar, M. S., & Warner, P. (1994). Selecting financial indices to measure critical path outcomes. *Nursing Management, 25*(9), 58-59.

Spath, P. (1995, August). How to manage your outcomes more effectively. *Hospital Peer Review, 8,* 120-124.

Wall, D. K., Joseph, E. D., & MacGrath, S. M. (1993). *Critical pathways: Development and implementation.* Chicago: Care Communications.

Wentworth, D. A., & Atkinson, R.P.M. (1996). Implementation of an acute stroke program decreases hospitalization costs and length of stay. *Stroke, 27*(6), 1040-1043.

Part III

Nursing Strategies in Community Settings

With the increase in managed health care organizations has come a decrease in the number of people who have affordable health care coverage. Also, the health care trends of recent years have resulted in a significant portion of health care services being delivered from community bases rather than from the acute-care hospital. Community agencies are predicted to be the source of growth for nursing employment. The increase in ambulatory care sites, community health centers, and home care settings has been extremely rapid during the transition from the fee-for-service era to the managed care era. Thus, nurses must learn to function in these new environments. The last section of this book will focus on nursing strategies in a variety of community settings.

Nurses have expressed serious concerns about the unequal distribution of health care services to the population. They are looking at new ways to increase services to the medically underserved. The use of advanced practice nurses in a variety of community settings is one way to meet these needs. Nurse case management services in community settings is a new strategy for such practice. Some recent permutations of this practice are in parish nursing, physician office practices, and entrepreneurial businesses. Case management as a strategy that focuses on a specific population will also be explored.

Another issue will be the role of the advanced practice nurse as an affordable alternative to the delivery of primary care. The use of nurse practitioners as primary care providers is continuing to escalate in the managed care environment. Examples of this use are included in this section of the book. The final chapter of the book provides a clinical example of a collaborative advanced nurse practice in a community health center.

Chapter

11

Nurse Case Management in Community Settings

Margaret M. Conger

There is an increasing recognition that non-traditional models of health care delivery must be considered and evaluated.

Barger and Rosenfeld (1993, p. 426)

Nurse case management within community settings is an area of growth. As length of hospital stay continues to shorten for patients, more people are returning to their homes in need of case management services. To meet this need, strategies used in acute-care hospital case management programs are being applied in a wide variety of community settings. Providing for continuity of services for clients using a variety of health care agencies located in communities is necessary. Timely provision of care so that resources are used in the most effective way is also important to manage the expenditure of health care dollars.

In this chapter, several community-based case management models will be described. It is impossible to discuss every outpatient setting in which case management occurs, but the models presented here will illustrate the application of case management principles. The reader can then apply these principles to another setting of interest. This chapter will look at case management issues relevant to long-term care, home-based programs, the parish nurse movement, and physician office group case management practices. These examples demonstrate the impact of nurse case management in community settings.

Long-Term Care

As the population in this country ages, there are increasing numbers of people who require health care on a long-term basis. This can be provided either in the home, with services such as home health nursing, or in institutions such as nursing homes. The elderly are often vulnerable to the changing priorities of the health care system because of their limited available financial and personal resources; they need an advocate to work through problems that arise as system changes occur. Often, public policy can be a hindrance to the person needing care. It is not uncommon for a person who needs help primarily with social service needs such as home health aide or a meals on wheels program to have to demonstrate a medical need (Shapiro, 1995). To "work the system," an unneeded medical intervention may be provided to meet criteria for care. Such practices lead to unnecessary use of health care resources.

The goal of long-term care is to aid functionally dependent persons without adequate resources to obtain needed health services to promote an optimal level of functioning (Shapiro, 1995). Nurse case management is a promising means to achieve this goal. Successful nurse case management programs have demonstrated effectiveness in facilitating the delivery of health care in a cost-effective manner. Examples of how this can be accomplished, both in an institutional setting such as a nursing home and in home-based programs, are provided here.

Nurse Case Management in a Nursing Home Setting

Development of nurse case management programs within a nursing home setting has been slow. Howe (1996) identifies a number of reasons for this. The limited number of registered nurses (RNs) employed in nursing home settings has been a deterrent. The majority of care provided in these institutions is by licensed practical nurses (LPNs) and nursing assistants (NAs). The use of large numbers of these lesser skilled nurses and assistants has led to a long tradition of task-oriented care, with little accountability for achieving predetermined outcomes. Nursing homes have also long been underfunded, receiving most of their financing from Medicaid or Medicare sources. Given these constraints, it is easy to see why the development of nurse case management programs in these settings has been very slow. Without professional nurses to spearhead changes in the care delivery system, and with little financial incentive to improve services, the development of nurse case management services is embryonic in nursing homes.

Despite these problems, the benefits to the residents of a nursing home from a nurse case management system can be tremendous (Howe, 1996). If a nurse develops a personalized plan of care based on specific resident needs, both the resident and family members will be more satisfied with the care. Benefits to staff members can also occur. A case management system in which the registered nurse works with a small group of assistive personnel to manage the care of a defined caseload can bring about positive changes in client-provider interactions. As each member of the team comes to know the residents within the care group as individuals, the interactions between the clients and the staff will lead to increased quality of care. As the quality of life for the resident is increased, the staff will develop greater satisfaction from their jobs.

The nurse case managers in the nursing home model described by Howe (1996) each took responsibility for up to seven residents and were responsible for serving as the liaison between the resident and the interdisciplinary care team. They reviewed each resident's chart to evaluate all medications, treatments, and other interventions and then developed an individualized care plan. Care plans were presented at interdisciplinary team meetings, which were held on a quarterly basis. Overall, each nurse case manager was held accountable for managing the needs of assigned residents. The nurse case manager also worked with specific nursing assistants who were permanently assigned to care for a small group of residents. The nursing assistants were responsible for managing the personal hygiene needs, dietary concerns, and other activities of daily living of the residents. This method of assignment was a radical departure from the former practice, in which the NAs were assigned to a different group of residents each shift, thus precluding development of personal relationships necessary to individualizing care.

Outcomes noted from this nurse case management program were increased resident satisfaction with their living situation and increased quality of life. Specific outcomes noted were a decrease in the rate of incontinence, less use of physical restraints, and an increase in the ability of residents to manage activities of daily living such as feeding and mobility. However, because of the expected decrease in functional ability of the residents due to the aging process, it is hard to quantify these outcomes. An unexpected finding was a decrease in the rate of staff turnover. Among the licensed staff, the rate dropped by 117%; among the NAs, the rate dropped by 229% following the introduction of nurse case management as the delivery system (Howe, 1996).

This example demonstrates that nursing case management can improve the quality of life in probably one of the most difficult living situations. Entry into a nursing home has long been viewed as the "end of the road." Any success in making this a more positive living environment is a credit to the nursing staff employed in these agencies.

Home-Based Programs

As patients are discharged from hospitals very early in their recovery from serious illness, need for care in the home has escalated, making home-based nursing one of the most rapidly growing fields of health care. This growth has led to a steep escalation of health care costs. An outcome of these increased costs is an attempt to strictly limit this care to those who are truly homebound. The Medicare definition for homebound is that the person is unable to leave the home except for limited visits to the physician's office or other essential business. Also, to qualify for home nursing care, the person must require frequent visits for treatments such as dressing changes, intravenous medications, or specialized teaching. As the client's health improves and such services are no longer needed, funding to provide home health care is eliminated.

Unfortunately, many of these clients and their caretakers still need considerable assistance with ongoing health and social needs. To meet this gap in care, nursing case management for homebound clients has arisen. The needs of these often elderly clients do not end when the acute medical problem is resolved. In fact, Helberg (1993) found that the ability of a person to function independently was more often related to nursing problems, functional status, and coping ability than to medical diagnosis. New ways to meet the needs of this group are needed. One organization, Carondelet St. Mary's in Tucson,

Arizona, has developed a model for home-based care that is widely copied throughout the country (Ethridge, 1991).

The Carondelet Experience

In response to the rapid shift in management of hospitalized patients that arose out of the movement into the prospective payment environment of the mid-1980s, the nursing management at Carondelet St. Mary's Hospital recognized a need for continued nursing care of discharged patients (Ethridge & Johnson, 1996; Michaels, 1992). Patients at high risk for hospital readmissions were found to be those who were frail, elderly, and had a chronic illness. Their retention of in-hospital teaching was low, leading to increased problems with self-management. However, many of these discharged patients did not meet criteria for home health nursing as defined by the Medicare guidelines. A need for a new type of nursing service was apparent. Out of these concerns was born the community nurse case management movement.

The Carondelet program provides services to persons who have a physiological imbalance, a cognitive deficit, or an emotional challenge. Problems that arise from caretaker issues can also be a reason for providing nurse case management services. If the person has no caretaker or if the caretaker has a knowledge deficit or is infirm, case management can be provided. Another problem that signals a need for inclusion in the program is that a person qualifies for home health services for a brief period but requires services following the end of home care coverage. Finally, persons who make frequent use of emergency departments or hospitals for immediate health care needs are targeted for possible nurse case management. The indicators for inclusion in the home-based nurse case management program are shown in Table 11.1.

The services provided include home visits for those clients who are unable to travel to community health centers, education for family and clients about symptom management and mediation or treatment use, and advocacy to obtain appropriate services needed in a timely fashion. The emphasis is placed on health promotion and disease prevention (Ethridge, 1991). The nurse case manager (NCM) monitors the client's health status, either through home or telephone visits, and coordinates both medical and community services as needed. An important part of the NCM role is to help the client build support networks with family members or friends. In 1990, a

TABLE 11.1 Criteria for Home-Based Nursing Case Management

Physiological imbalance
Cognitive deficit
Emotionally challenged
Has no caretaker
Has a caretaker with a knowledge deficit
Has a caretaker who is infirm
Qualifies for limited home health services for a brief period but requires additional services
Demonstrated pattern of frequent use of emergency room or hospital for immediate health care needs

community-based capitated program was begun, using a nursing HMO as the organizational framework (Ethridge & Johnson, 1996). Under this system, each enrolled person paid $2.20 per month as a part of the HMO premium for community health nursing services. The client was matched with the level of service that the nurse case manager determined would be most effective. These ranged from the most acute hospice care through a spectrum including home nurse case management to services provided in nursing community centers. The desired outcome of the case management services was an increase in each client's ability to manage self-care. If the enrollee required care within the hospital, the NCM would follow his or her progress, actively plan for discharge, and subsequently monitor all community services needed.

The outcomes of this nurse case management program have been impressive. Because of the frequent nurse monitoring, deterioration in a client's chronic condition has been picked up early and managed either by an outpatient visit to a physician or admission to the hospital at a lower level of acuity than had been previously seen. Fewer of these people were admitted to critical care units, thus saving the hospital large amounts of money. Also, when a hospital admission was necessary, the stay tended to be shorter than prior to the nurse case management program (Ethridge & Johnson, 1996).

Outcomes achieved under the nursing HMO have attracted national attention. Review of the program indicates a high level of satisfaction among the clients, increased ability to manage symptoms of chronic conditions, and increased self-care abilities. Financially, the program has been successful. There have been a reduced number of emergency department visits and fewer hospital admissions among the enrollees. Data from the first year of service under the nursing HMO show that the number of admissions to the hospital from this group was 1,311 per 1,000 enrollees. The national average from other Medicare HMO programs at the same time was over 1,800 per 1,000 enrollees (Ethridge & Johnson, 1996).

Parish Nursing

Parish nursing is a type of community-based nurse case management that has arisen in the United States. Although a parish nurse program is rarely associated with a managed care organization, it is a service that is becoming more necessary as a result of fewer services being offered by managed care organizations. Thus, it is an area to consider as one thinks about the effects managed care has had on nursing practice. There are probably several factors important to the rapid increase in parish nursing programs. Interest in preventive health practices and health promotion activities has grown as more people have come to realize that health care costs are out of control. Also, as people become more aware of the spiritual influences on health, there is increased demand for such services. The rise in holistic health practices has been an important factor in the increased interest in parish nurse programs.

Parish nurse ministry began in the Chicago area under the influence of Granger Westberg, a Lutheran pastor who had many years of experience working as a chaplain in large medical centers. During his work as a hospital chaplain, he was able to bring doctors, nurses, chaplains, and patients together to explore the spiritual dimensions of illness. One of the needs that quickly became apparent was a greater focus on preventive health measures that could reduce the incidence of serious medical problems. Soon, some experimental health centers were established in local churches where physicians, nurses, and pastors worked cooperatively to help people manage their health. Westberg (1990) found that nurses were excellent catalysts to get physicians and pastors to talk with each other.

The movement to place nurses within local parishes rapidly spread to hundreds of congregations across the county. Westberg (1990) describes the ideal parish nurse as a person who is spiritually mature and sensitive to the relationship between faith and health and its application to spiritual aspects of health care. The work of each parish nurse is shaped by the needs of the specific congregation served, but there are several underlying principles that are applicable to all congregations. The aim of the program is to provide holistic wellness through integration of faith and health.

Most parish nurse programs are under the direction of a Health Cabinet that includes individuals concerned with the health needs of members of the congregations. This group is usually instrumental in bringing a parish nurse into the congregation. Bergquist and King (1994) have identified four general areas of practice for the parish nurse. These are health educator, health counselor, leader of individuals and groups, and community liaison. These roles are very similar to those previously identified for the nurse case manager. In addition, Westberg (1990) emphasizes the need for the parish nurse to always keep the close relationship between faith and health central to the members of the congregation. Each of these roles will be discussed in more detail.

Health Educator

The health educator role is a primary function of the parish nurse. Education can occur in one-on-one sessions with a member of the congregation on a specific health issue or with larger groups on health topics of general interest. Topics often included in this kind of education concern self-help, such as parenting skills, cardiopulmonary resuscitation techniques, weight management, stress reduction, and general health management. Dependent upon the needs of the local congregation, classes on specific health problems are also offered. Because the parish nurse is aware of the health problems of members of the congregation, specific education classes can be developed based on interests generated from these problems. For example, if a member has a myocardial infarction, this would be an excellent time to educate the congregation on lifestyle changes important to the prevention of heart disease.

Health Counselor

The health counselor role is a integral part of the parish nurse role. Counseling can cover topics such as physical, emotional, social, or spiritual concerns (Bergquist & King, 1994).

The parish nurse is often sought out by members of the congregation to discuss personal problems. Also, the nurse will make visits to members of the congregation in their homes, hospital, or long-term care facility. Families often seek out the parish nurse for assistance in making decisions about safety and living arrangements for the elderly (Djupe, 1996).

Leader of Groups and Individuals

Leadership in the congregation is an important part of the parish nurse's activity. The task of working with the health needs of all persons in a congregation is greater than what one person can usually manage. Thus developing volunteers to work with the program is important. The parish nurse uses the skills of members of the congregation to assist in activities such as health fairs, immunization clinics, and self-help groups.

Community Liaison

It is in the realm of community liaison that the parish nurse most closely resembles the nurse case manager. Referrals to community agencies, health organizations, and physicians are an important part of the work of the parish nurse. The parish nurse must become familiar with community agencies so that these relationships are fostered. In a pilot program in Iowa, parish nurses and community health nurses teamed together to foster the health of community members (King, Lakin, & Striepe, 1993). One kind of collaborative activity that has been developed is that of reciprocal referrals between public health nurses and parish nurses. The parish nurses, with their familiarity with the members of local congregations, have been helpful to the public health nurses in identifying community members with specific health needs. The public health nurses have also supplied the parish nurses with health literature that is available at the county level. The two groups of nurses also collaborated in providing educational and screening programs.

Spiritual Care

In the realm of spiritual care, the parish nurse works in conjunction with the ministerial staff of the church to assist members of the congregation to integrate faith and well being. This is often accomplished by working with individuals and families in crisis. The nurse's spiritual concern is demonstrated by listening to the client's story and answering questions. The person may need spiritual counseling to develop insight into and understanding of the problem. The emphasis is always placed on helping people better understand the mind, body, and spirit interconnection.

Organization of a Parish Nurse Program

Several models have been developed for organizing a parish nurse program. In some programs, the parish nurse is recruited and employed directly by the local congregation. There are also programs in which the local congregation contracts with a nurse to provide volunteer service to carry out the work of parish nursing. In both of these situations, the parish nurse is advised to network with other parish nurses to gain consultation and resources needed to carry out the work. The Nurse Ministries Network (1997) in Phoenix, Arizona, provides such services to parish nurses, both in the Phoenix area and statewide. The network provides both initial training and ongoing support for parish nurses. After initial training, the nurses move out into their assigned congregations to carry out their work and then meet as a group at least monthly to support each other in their ministry.

In other models, the parish nurse is connected to a hospital or other health agency and is then contracted out to the local congregation. This is the model that was initially begun by Westberg (1990) through the Lutheran General Health System. The health organization funded the parish nurse and provided education and resources for the nurses. The local congregations then provided office facilities for the nurse. The cost of the parish nurse salary was jointly shared by the local congregation and the agency. An important aspect of both of these models is the need for a structure to provide for education, emotional and resource support, and consultative services for the parish nurse.

Within each congregation, a support group (frequently called a health cabinet) is formed to oversee the health-related activities of the church. The parish nurse is a member of this group but is not in charge of it. Westberg (1990) suggests that any church considering the development of a parish nurse program first form such a cabinet. The function of the health cabinet is to oversee and support the work of the parish nurse. The working out of the relationship between the parish nurse and the health cabinet becomes an individual process. Often, members of the health cabinet can take over some of the organizational activities to support the various health projects developed. They serve as a true support service to the parish nurse, who otherwise could become overwhelmed with the multiple needs of the members of the congregation. Persons within the congregation who have a vision for a health ministry are logical choices for membership on this cabinet. The presence of people with some health background such as physicians, nurses, dentists, allied health workers, and health educators is valuable for this committee.

Physician Office Case Management

An innovative area for case management that is emerging is the physician office, particularly in those groups associated with managed care organizations. Many persons living in the community are finding it more difficult to deal with the highly fragmented health care and social systems present in this country. This is particularly true of the elderly population. Assistance with finding solutions to managing chronic health conditions is a needed service, and many look to their physicians for help. However, physicians are trained to diagnose and treat disease conditions but are not prepared to deal with the multitude of problems associated with chronic illness. Thus, there is a need for a health care professional to work alongside the physician and assist with such management.

Several models for such services have been reported in the literature. White, Gundrum, Shearer, and Simmons (1994) report on the model developed at Huntington Memorial Hospital in Pasadena, California. In this model, social workers who are knowledgeable about community resources have been hired by a senior care network that provides services for a large elderly group of clients to link the physician's office with community resources. They function in a case management role to assist clients with health-related problems.

Clients are referred to the case managers by the physician, an office staff person, or through identification of specific needs revealed through the use of a questionnaire given to the clients as they come for office visits. The questionnaire focuses on issues such as frequent use of the hospital or emergency department, changes in living arrangements, difficulties with activities in daily living, care provider problems, or problems with sleep, vision, or depression (White et al., 1994). Often, office staff members will identify a potential candidate for case management services because the client may frequently miss physician appointments, be behind in making financial payments, or ask for assistance with a problem.

The case manager makes contact with potential clients either directly in the physician's office, through a phone call, or, often, during a home visit. A complete assessment of both the client and the living arrangement is made. Often, psychological problems as well as social problems are identified that require a community agency referral. Common needs identified are for social services such as transportation, adult day care arrangements, new housing arrangements, or financial services. The case manager often becomes involved in helping clients secure durable medical items such as a hospital bed, mobilization equipment, or assistive devices. Most interactions between the case manager and the client are short term, with the identified problem being managed within two to three visits.

Another program in which case management services are provided within the context of physician's offices is the St. Joseph's Healthcare System in Albuquerque, New Mexico (Anker-Unnever & Netting, 1995). This is a managed care group that provides services to a large elderly population. The physicians had identified the need for a means to monitor patients in their homes and to assess compliance with ordered medication and treatment regimens. They also recognized a need for someone to arrange for community health and social service needs for their clients. Arranging for transportation back and forth to health care services was also seen as a need.

In this model, both social workers and nurses are used as case managers and work in conjunction with several large physician groups. The case managers developed a screening tool for identifying clients who were at high risk for problems in managing chronic health needs. Identifiers included an age of 65 years or older with a chronic illness such as congestive heart failure, postcerebral vascular accident, diabetes, respiratory disease, or a hip fracture. However, as the program developed, physicians found clients with a number of other conditions whom they felt would benefit from case management services. Problems that arose from a lack of family or caregiver support, history of frequent hospitalizations, nutritional deficits, memory or judgment problems, frequent falls, or noncompliance with the physician treatment plan also became triggers for case management referrals. The need for case management services was closely tied to the person's need for nursing care rather than an outcome of a particular disease. This finding is similar to that found by Helberg (1993). She noted that a patient's need for nursing services was more closely related to functional status, coping abilities, and presence of nursing problems than to a medical diagnosis.

The model for this case management program is one of brokerage; that is, monitoring of general health needs and referral services rather than direct in-home care services. However, some simple physiological monitoring such as blood pressure checking is also done. The need for more in-depth home monitoring is under discussion.

Conclusions

In reviewing these programs, it can be seen that providing case management services in community settings is a growing field for nurses. As the elderly population increases, more case management programs will need to be developed. The models for nurse case management in a variety of community settings presented in this chapter provide direction for the future of nursing practice. As the pressure for increased cost efficiency and appropriate resource utilization continues to grow, increased amounts of health care will be provided in settings outside of the acute-care hospital. The old paradigm in which the majority of nursing care was delivered within a hospital setting is rapidly disappearing. The time has come for nurses to learn a new way to practice in the new managed care health environment.

Community-based nursing is an exciting challenge for nursing. Much of the care provided in this setting focuses on health promotion and disease prevention, areas in which nurses have always been expert. Because of nurses' ability to assist people to manage both the physical and social problems associated with chronic illness, they make ideal health care providers. As managed care organizations take on a larger market share of health care, there will be increased opportunities for nurse case managers in community settings. This is a return to nursing's roots in such community-based programs as the Henry Street Settlement House in New York or the Frontier Nursing service in Kentucky. The ideals of the public health nurse making a difference in the community are once again being activated.

References

Anker-Unnever, L., & Netting, F. E. (1995). Coordinated care partnership: Case management with physician practices. *Journal of Case Management, 4*(1), 3-8.

Barger, S., & Rosenfeld, P. (1993). Models in community health care. *Nursing and Health Care, 14*(8), 426-431.

Bergquist, S., & King, J. (1994). Parish nursing: A conceptual framework. *Journal of Holistic Nursing, 12*(2), 155-170.

Djupe, A. M. (1996). Parish nursing. In E. L. Cohen (Ed.), *Nurse case management in the 21st century* (pp. 211-221). St. Louis, MO: Mosby.

Ethridge, P. (1991). A nursing HMO: Carondelet St. Mary's experience. *Nursing Management, 22*(7), 22-27.

Ethridge, P., & Johnson, S. (1996). The influence of reimbursement on nurse case management practice: Carondelet's experience. In E. L. Cohen (Ed.), *Nurse case management in the 21st century* (pp. 245-255). St. Louis, MO: Mosby.

Helberg, J. L. (1993). Patient's status at home discharge. *Image: The Journal of Nursing Scholarship, 25*(2), 93-99.

Howe, S. R. (1996). Nurse case management and long-term care. In E. L. Cohen (Ed.), *Nurse case management in the 21st century* (pp. 149-155). St. Louis, MO: Mosby.

King, J. M., Lakin, J. A., & Striepe, J. (1993). Coalition building between public health nurses and parish nurses. *Journal of Nursing Administration, 23*(2), 27-31.

Michaels, C. (1992). Carondelet St. Mary's nursing enterprise. *Nursing Clinics of North America, 27*(1), 77-85.

Nurse Ministries Network. (1997). *Parish nurse resource manual.* Phoenix, AZ: Author.

Shapiro, E. (1995). Case-management in long-term care. *Journal of Case Management, 4*(2), 43-47.

Westberg, G. E. (1990). *The parish nurse: Providing a minister of health for your congregation.* Minneapolis, MN: Augsburg/Fortress.

White, M., Gundrum, G., Shearer, S., & Simmons, W. (1994, June). A role for case managers in the physician office. *Journal of Case Management, 3*(2), 62-68.

Chapter

12

Population-Based Nurse Case Management

Margaret M. Conger

The greatest good for the greatest number of people.
Shamansky (1995) (and others)

As health care costs continue to escalate, even within the managed care environment, new ways to provide care in a cost-effective manner are being sought. One such newly emerging trend in health care agencies is to develop case management services that focus on a specific population that uses similar services. It has been found that by committing specific members of the health care team to concentrate their efforts with this population, the quality of care can be enhanced and health care costs can be reduced. This type of model is called population-based case management.

Population-based case management requires the provider to take a broader perspective than that needed when working individual patients. The planning of care must move to a focus on how the needs of the entire group can be met. It is based on the public health maxim of the "greatest good for the greatest number of people" (Shamansky, 1995, p. 212). Because most nurses have been educated to look at the good of the individual, a shift in thinking is necessary for nurses to be effective in this new strategy. They need a new vision to see that by doing good for the entire group, the needs of the individual will be maximized. This type of thinking has not been a part of the socialization of the nurse in the past, but it is necessary to deal with the economic realities of the managed care environment.

Population-Based Case Management

Because of the high costs associated with treating poorly managed chronic health conditions such as diabetes, many health maintenance organizations (HMOs) are beginning to focus on a population-based case management as a strategy to deliver health care. The goal for such a program is to maximize the health outcomes of this population and reduce the cost of its care by assuring that the care provided is effective. Also, many of the services that public health programs have provided in the past are being shifted to managed care organizations (Primomo, 1995). For example, child immunization programs, once largely the responsibility of public health agencies, now are managed by the HMO. Other examples include screening for health conditions such as hypertension, diabetes, or other chronic diseases.

Nurses working in managed care organizations must either learn or relearn public health skills to be effective in this environment. One way to do this is to focus on specific populations, such as those with a chronic illness, or an age group such as the pediatric population.

To assist nurses in understanding the differences in health care delivery from this perspective, the issues of population-based case management will be explored. This chapter will look at a variety of population-based case management programs that are geared to a specific population based on age groups. This theme will be continued in the next chapter, where the population will be defined by special health needs related to disease-specific or environmental conditions.

Methods Used in Population-Based Case Management

The first step in developing a population-based case management program is to identify the target population. To do this, a review of the demographics of the organization in which you are working must be done. The subpopulation should represent a significant percentage of the population of the HMO or should require a considerable percentage of the provider's cost. It is important to the success of the eventual outcome measurement process to have a large enough population using similar services, so aggregate data can be collected. Another factor to consider when selecting the target population is how a program devised for this group can be evaluated. The selected population should be able to respond to the clinical interventions selected, and these responses must be significant enough so that differences in outcome measures can be observed (Shamansky, 1995).

After the subpopulation has been selected, the next step is to develop protocols appropriate for the management of this group. Only those monitoring elements and treatment modalities that have been shown to be effective should be included. A review of the literature will help in sorting out effective management practices from those based only in tradition. In some agencies, these protocols are developed as a clinical pathway similar to those used in acute-care hospital settings (Primomo, 1995).

Tools to monitor the outcomes of the care and to evaluate treatments also need to be developed. This is a strategic point in population-based case management because of the need to validate the effectiveness of the health care strategies used. Use of resources on ineffective treatments, when provided to a large group, will quickly lead to escalation of costs. One advantage of using population-based case management is that data are collected from a large group and can then be used to evaluate patterns of practice. This is an important key to cost-effective practice.

For example, if working with a subpopulation of persons with diabetes, treatment strategies such as educational programs or counseling and coaching sessions, as well as more traditional treatments using medications and dietary instructions, must all be examined as to their effectiveness. What "nurse dose," or time spent with a nurse, is needed to aid patients with a chronic illness such as diabetes maintain control of blood sugar levels? What is the cost benefit of frequent nurse-client interactions to help a person with diabetes make lifestyle changes that will result in the reduction of complications such as blindness, kidney failure, or the need for the amputation of a limb? Answers to questions like these cannot be found when working with individual clients. However, when working with the larger group, it should be possible to determine effective patterns of practice. Research in the area of effective nursing interventions when providing population-based care is an exciting opportunity for nursing. The population selected can be based on a variety of circumstances such as living environment, specific disease, or age. Both the very young child and the elderly pose special problems for health care that make these groups ideal for such a program. Pregnant young adults form another subgroup that is responsive to nursing interventions and whose increased health can make a significant impact on reducing health care expenditures. Examples of programs serving special populations will be presented in this chapter to illustrate how case management principles can be applied to special populations.

Case Management Based on Living Circumstances

New interest is arising in looking at subpopulations based on living circumstances, particularly groups such as the homeless or migrant groups. These populations usually fall outside the realm of the typical managed care organization because they have no employer-sponsored health coverage. However, as state programs for the medically indigent increase, these populations are being covered by a capitated managed care plan. In states such as Arizona, Hawaii, and Tennessee, the Medicaid program is set up using managed care organizations to serve the health needs of this population. However, even though provision is often available for health care, the special circumstances of this population often preclude their accessing it. Thus, an active case management program that specializes in serving the needs of this population is important.

The homeless population in this country is rapidly growing, with an increased number of families with children (Wagner & Menke, 1992). A similar increase in the migrant population is also occurring (Good, 1992). The health care needs of both the homeless and migrant populations are staggering. Community resources tend to be fragmented, making it difficult for these families to access even the services that are available. Health care that is accessed tends to be on an emergency basis; thus the cost for care that is used is at the most expensive end of the health care spectrum. The amount of mental illness and substance abuse among this population tends to be much higher than that found in the general population. Also, the unstable living conditions are often associated with problems with nutrition, dental care, and deficiencies in the immune system, making these people very vulnerable to infectious diseases (Good, 1992; Wagner & Menke, 1992). Social needs are acute, with an obvious immediate need for housing; the need for food to provide adequate nutrition follows a close second.

In the face of the many problems presented by homeless or migrant families, case management programs are needed to assist this population to achieve a higher level of health. The case manager must develop a personal relationship with the client because these persons have had a long history of distrust of government services. Also, because of the specific nature of each population, the program must be designed around the needs for that population. Programs that focus on providing clinical services as well as brokering services have been shown to be most successful (Mercier & Racine, 1995).

Services that need to be included in a case management program include provision of health care, either direct or through referral to local agencies, support in living arrangements (i.e., food and housing), and emotional support to assist clients to manage the multitude of problems they bring with them to the present situation. A number of clients also need assistance in developing independent living skills.

Examples of programs that have been successful in working with these populations demonstrate that nurse case management can have a positive impact on the lives of these people. Wagner and Menke (1992) worked with homeless families in Columbus, Ohio to assist them with both health and social needs. They worked out of a neighborhood center, using a brokering model; that is, they referred clients to other agencies rather than providing direct care themselves. One important agency that was the first referral for many of the clients was a shelter for homeless women and children. Clients in need of medical care were referred to a community health service. A unique program that they worked with was one that paired elderly residents needing companions with young homeless persons. Through this program, they were able to move some of their clients into stable living arrangements.

Good (1992) found that a program that provided a clinical service—a school-based dental health management program—served as an access to migrant families. Through the contacts made in the dental program, the need for additional services was identified and the program expanded to include health teaching and management of social issues. As families became comfortable with the nurse case manager through the dental clinic, they were willing to seek out her assistance for other health issues.

Case management among homeless or migrant families requires holistic care to be able to problem solve with families who have few resources to meet the needs of everyday life. Both strong clinical skills and knowledge of the services provided by social agencies are necessary to be effective with this group. Because the needs of this population are specialized, the nursing interventions must be unique. Nurses with a strong basis in holistic health care have demonstrated that they can positively affect the health of this population.

Case Management of Special-Needs Infants

Case management programs to work with young children with special health needs are rapidly increasing following passage of the Education for the Handicapped Act (PL 99-457, 1986; Federal Register, 1989) by the federal government. One provision in this act requires that a qualified health care professional assume case management activities for children with special health needs such as cerebral palsy, congenital defects affecting any of the body organs, Down syndrome, or any other physical or mental condition that can affect the child's development.

The responsibilities of the case manager in this program are to work with the family to assist them in decision-making skills and to empower them to work within the complex health care system. The nurse case manager is also expected to conduct a comprehensive needs assessment and contribute information to the health care team as the plan of care is developed. Coordination of services is also extremely important so that both the time and effort of the parents, as well as that of the health care team, is used effectively. The nurse case manager is also expected to monitor the progress of the infant and family (Steele, 1991). Perhaps the most important role for the case manager is that of counselor and coach for the family as they struggle with the multitude of problems that a special needs child can present. This support is vital to the family so that it can maintain its stability and continue to function as the caregiver. Without it, many families may find the burden of care too heavy and seek some type of institutionalized care for the child, at a greatly increased cost.

Common problems that have been identified in families with infants with special needs include difficulty in obtaining the basic necessities of life (poverty), lack of transportation, functional illiteracy, and lack of emotional and informational resources (Poland, Giblin, Waller, & Bayer, 1991). It is not uncommon for problems such as these to become so overwhelming that the family can no longer focus on the needs of the infant, and the family then drops out of the intervention program (Steele, 1991). Thus, the support of the case manager in helping families find solutions to these problems will bring benefit to the child.

In the Parent-Infant Enrichment program described by Steele (1991), development of parent group meetings was very effective in assisting parents to develop problem-solving skills. Sharing successes and failures with other parents provided a forum for individual parent learning. It also provided an emotional support group because of the sense that all the parents were facing similar problems. The parents were able to help each other through the "rough times" far more effectively than could a health professional who had not faced the same problems.

Coordination of services was also extremely important. Parents needed a lot of encouragement to get all of the required health screening done for the child to be eligible for public-funded services. They needed assistance in filling out forms and getting the necessary appointments to establish the need for care. The nurse case manager also worked with the health care providers to guide them through completing all of the necessary paperwork. Often these providers were not familiar with the requirements to meet all of the government mandates. When an experienced nurse case manager guided them through the process, the paperwork was done correctly the first time, saving much frustration both for the provider and the parents.

Using a nurse as the case manager rather than a social worker proved to be very helpful because, although social service problems were often very important, education about health care needs was also needed. The nurse was able to provide instruction on how to handle the health problems normally experienced by infants as well as those problems specific to the disease condition. Teaching the families to manage these minor health care situations was an important way in which health care costs could be reduced.

This program demonstrated that nurses had both the clinical and communications skills required to be effective in working with families who had children with special health care needs. The families were supported as they tried to achieve optimal functioning for their children. The nurses developed expert skills in problem solving with this group through repeated experiences with similar problems. This level of expertise would have been difficult to develop if the nurse worked with a wide variety of clients rather than a specific population.

Case Management of High-Risk Pregnancy

Another group that has great potential for a reduction in health care costs through nurse case management is high-risk pregnant women. Because the costs of caring for preterm infants is enormous, money spent to bring these women to a full-term pregnancy will be saved many times over. Women identified as high risk because of tobacco, alcohol, or drug use also need the services of a case manager. Reducing the incidence of an infant born with fetal alcohol syndrome or addicted to a drug will provide long-term cost savings both to the health care organization and to community social service agencies. Such education is actually best provided prior to the time of conception to achieve the greatest effect and should be a part of all managed care organizations.

One program designed to increase the health of pregnant women was through the Carondelet St. Mary's Nursing Network (Ethridge & Johnson, 1996). A contract to manage the health needs of high-risk pregnant women was negotiated with the Arizona Health Care Cost Containment System (AHCCCS), Arizona's Medicaid system, which functions as a capitated organization to provide health care for the poor. This program included education aimed at reducing the use of tobacco, alcohol, and drug use as well as services to women identified as having a preterm delivery.

Case management of women at high risk for a preterm infant has been shown to be extremely cost-effective (More & Mandell, 1997). Every day that the pregnancy can be extended increases the likelihood of delivering a healthy infant. Often these women are ordered to maintain bed rest for considerable periods of time, even though the family situation may make this very difficult to follow through on. The case manager is needed to assist the client and family with finding a way to follow this order. The cost of short-term homemaker care is far less than the cost of caring for the premature infant (More & Mandell, 1997). However, it often requires the negotiation skills of an experienced case manager to make this case with the insurance organization and obtain funding for this needed service.

Case Management of the Elderly

The population in the United States is aging at an unprecedented rate in human history. In 1996, the number of people age 65 years or older was 8 times greater than in 1900, but the number of people 75 to 84 years old was 16 times larger and the number of people 85 or older was 31 times larger (American Association of Retired Persons [AARP], 1997). Nationally, people age 65 or older comprise 13.1% of the population. If the increase continues as expected, by the year 2020 about 20% of the population of the United States will be 65 years old or older (AARP, 1997). With increasing age come increasing chronic health concerns. Approximately 50% of all people age 65 have arthritis in one or more joints, 36% have high blood pressure, 32% have heart disease, 17% have cataracts, and 10% have diabetes (AARP, 1997). Nationally, 53.9% of all older people have trouble with mobility or self-care, but as seen in Table 12.1, assistance needs increase rapidly with advancing age.

These alterations in health status are associated with limitations in a person's ability to manage either household activities such as shopping or preparing meals or do self-care activities such as bathing and dressing. These needs of the geriatric population make this group an excellent focus for nurse case management services. However, the type of services required will vary from one age segment of this population to another. Those who are fully functional, that is, who are able to live independently, may only need assistance in managing a chronic illness. Others, who tend to be in the older cohort of the elderly, have limited functional ability and require assistance with managing activities of daily living. This group will require a greater array of services. Age is not the only factor that will determine the level of care that any one person requires, but the data support the point that the percentage of the elderly requiring assistance increases markedly with age. When developing case management programs, these differences in need must be considered.

Health Care System Limitations

The American health care system has traditionally focused on meeting acute-care needs. This system does not serve the needs of the elderly population well because this population's needs tend to be related to chronic health problems. The focus on acute care has resulted in resource-intensive care centered around hospital services, but funding for services that will keep the elderly well in the community has not been available (Moneyham & Scott, 1997). Many of the services needed by the elderly are not reimbursable under most health insurance plans. For example, Medicare health insurance, which is the major insurer of older Americans, does not pay for assistance once an

TABLE 12.1 Degree of Need for Assistance Correlated With Age

Age Group	*Percentage Needing Assistance*
65-69	7.3
70-74	11.9
75-84	22.5
85+	42.3

SOURCE: Adapted from Adams and Marano (1994).

acute episode of illness has passed or once a person is unable to continue to make progress toward independent living. New approaches to health care funding are needed to meet the needs of the geriatric population.

Need for Case Management Services

Preliminary studies are beginning to demonstrate that active case management of this group can have a significant impact on reducing use of services and, thus, cost (Ethridge, 1991; Ethridge & Johnson, 1996; Michaels, 1992; Pierini, 1988). Scott and Rantz (1997) suggest that providing the necessary support and improving the self-management skills of this population is the key to providing cost-effective health care.

The case management needs of this group can be organized into medical, functional, and social areas. Medical needs include assistance with interventions such as medication usage, information about health conditions, monitoring and management of chronic health conditions, guidance with appropriate use of medical services, and actual nursing interventions such as wound care or assistance with incontinence problems. Functional problems include issues of mobility, developing self-care capabilities, brokering for needed support services, and coordinating care providers. Social needs include ways to reduce the social isolation often experienced by this group and assistance in developing coping mechanisms to deal with the multiple losses experienced.

A model for nurse case management of a geriatric population has been developed by Scott and Rantz (1997). In this model, the nurse case manager works actively with the primary provider and the health system as a whole to advocate for the services that will increase the client's self-management skills.

The nurse case manager must actively work with the client and family to develop a trust relationship to be effective. If the nurse case manager is able to reduce barriers to the client's optimal functioning and needed services are provided, the use of health care resources can be reduced.

Outcome measures for evaluating the success of a nurse case management program for a geriatric population have been identified (Scott & Rantz, 1997). The need for quality care that is cost effective remains paramount. The cost effectiveness of the care can be measured by determining the emergency and acute-care services used prior to the introduction of nurse case management services. Another important outcome to be evaluated for this population is access to care. Because of the place-bound limitations these clients often experience, access to care can become very difficult. The third area for evaluation is the reported well-being of the clients. This can be measured by determining their functional ability, the stabilization of physical symptoms, the amount of self-management they are able to maintain, and, finally, personal and family satisfaction. The indicators are shown in Table 12.2.

Services: Functionally Independent Elderly

A model that can be used for serving the health needs of the elderly who are able to function independently in the community is that of community health centers. Such centers have been established in senior centers, retirement complexes, churches, and low-income housing projects. Their goal is to provide nursing services in locations where community residents can conveniently obtain primary health care. The types of services offered include both acute care and chronic care, including monitoring and management for chronic conditions. Health teaching and health promotion activities such as nutritional counseling, medication teaching, stress reduction, management of lifestyle changes, and exercise promotion are also offered. Finally, the nurses provide assistance with accessing community resources.

One example of such a model is found in Tucson, Arizona (Michaels, 1992), with the Carondelet Health System, in which a number of health centers have been established in community halls in retirement villages, mobile home parks, and churches. Most of these centers are open for 4-hour periods once or twice a week. These centers serve the elderly who are mobile within their community. A special population served by these centers are those who come from a home base in the colder parts of the country to the Southwest

TABLE 12.2 Outcome Indicators for Geriatric Nurse Case Management Services

- Quality care
- Cost-effective care measured by decrease in use of emergency and acute-care services
- Convenient access to care
- Client well-being
    - Functional ability
    - Stabilization of physical symptoms
    - Amount of self-management skills
    - Personal and family satisfaction

to spend the winter. In this travel, they leave behind their primary health care providers. Those enrolled in a managed care organization have a great deal of difficulty in seeking alternate providers in the temporary location. With no established health service in the new community, this population has not had a place to go for symptom monitoring. This lack of health care can lead to relatively minor health problems escalating into major problems, resulting in the need for hospitalization.

The establishment of community health centers has been demonstrated to be quite effective. For example, Ethridge (1991) reports a noticeable decline in the acuity of patients admitted to the hospital with problems stemming from diabetes management since the health centers have been operational. Clients are having their blood sugar levels checked at the health center and are being referred for management before acute problems occur. The monitoring accomplished at the health centers has resulted in significant cost savings.

Another example of a nurse-managed wellness center is reported by Resick, Taylor, Carroll, D'Antonio, and Chesnay (1997). This center was established in a federally subsidized high-rise apartment in an inner city community. The clinic is staffed by a nurse practitioner and various nursing and allied health students from a nearby university and is held in a room near the building's activity center; it is thus readily accessible to the residents.

Most of the residents were eligible for Medicare health coverage and had a primary physician, but they still had many health concerns. These included the need for blood pressure monitoring; education about medications, diet, and exercise; and an arm-chair exercise program. The most common health concerns were the management of chronic illnesses such as diabetes mellitus, heart disease, pulmonary disease, and hypertension. Psychiatric problems, particularly depression, were also reported. Problems arising out of these medical conditions were impaired mobility, arthritis, amputations, and foot care needs.

The primary nursing services offered were monitoring of chronic health problems and health education. Examples of positive outcomes of the program were many. The nurse was able to assist one client who was incorrectly taking a heart medication in reducing his dosage before he got into serious trouble. She was also able to recognize impending pulmonary congestion in a resident with congestive heart failure and get her an immediate admission to the hospital for treatment. Thus, even in a population that theoretically had access to disease care, having a nurse in close proximity meant markedly improved health status.

Services: Limited-Function Elderly

The number of persons who require assistance with both health care needs and activities of daily living is increasing in that population older than 75 years (see Table 12.1). New services are needed to assist this population with limited functional ability to remain within the community. Some have family members living nearby who can assist with their care. Others live in group homes within the community.

A model for case management service to those elderly persons living in a group home is the practice of D. Lewis, RN, MS (Personal communication, March, 1998). Ms. Lewis contracts her services to adult day care homes that provide care for 6 to 10 elderly residents. The caregivers in these homes are usually certified nursing assistants (CNAs) and noncertified caregivers with little formal training in the care of the elderly. The services provided by Ms. Lewis include development of an individualized care plan for each resident that must be updated every 3 months, education and role modeling for the CNAs, and assessment of changing client needs. The adult day care provider is billed for all services. This practice is an example of an entrepreneurial nursing effort that is becoming more common as advanced practice nurses move out into the community and develop businesses that provide needed nursing skills.

Another model for case management services for elderly persons with limited function has been developed by the Carondelet Health Services and is widely copied throughout the country (Ethridge, 1991). This service was discussed in detail in Chapter 11. The Carondelet program provides services to persons who have a physiological imbalance, a cognitive deficit, or an emotional challenge. An important part of this service is provision of support for family caregivers, which enables the family to cope with the demands of caring for a frail elderly person.

With the provision of these services, elderly persons with limited functional ability have been able to remain in their homes rather than seeking care in long-term care facilities, thus both improving the quality of life and significantly reducing health care expenditures.

A home-based program for the chronically ill elderly is reported by Boyd, Fisher, Davidson, and Neilsen (1996). In this program, the nurse case managers worked with specific physician groups to assist clients discharged from a community hospital with a chronic illness. The type of services offered included the following:

- Assessment of needs
- Development of the plan of care
- Referral and coordination of resources
- Medication and symptom management
- Crisis intervention
- Liaison for patient and caregiver with health care personnel
- Counseling services

This study demonstrated a significant difference in health care resource utilization between the case-managed study group and the control group that did not receive case management services. The number of hospital admissions, emergency department visits, and primary care visits were all lower than in the control group. The authors also concluded that because of the decreased need for hospitalization, the quality of life of the case-managed group was improved.

Conclusions

The skills of advanced practice nurses working with specific populations are a welcome addition to communities in need of nursing services. A nurse who is knowledgeable about the needs of a specific population can make important contributions to the health of that population. Working with aggregates rather than the individual will lead to accumulation of rich data to support the effectiveness of these services. Such case management services have been shown to be effective in reducing the need for costly health expenditures and providing for increased quality of life of the recipients of the service. The future growth potential for nursing case management services aimed at specific populations is excellent.

References

American Association of Retired Persons. (1997). *A profile of older Americans*. Washington, DC: Author.

Adams, P. F., & Marano, M. A. (1994). Current estimates from the National Health Interview Survey, 1994. *National Center for Health Statistics, Vital Health Statistics, 10*(193), 83-84.

Boyd, M. L., Fisher, B., Davidson, A. W., & Neilsen, C. A. (1996). Community-based case management for chronically ill older adults. *Nursing Management, 27*(11), 31-32.

Education for the Handicapped Act, Pub. L. No. 99-487. (1991).

Ethridge, P. (1991). A nursing HMO: Carondelet St. Mary's experience. *Nursing Management, 22*(7), 22-27.

Ethridge, P., & Johnson, S. (1996). The influence of reimbursement on nurse case management practice: Carondelet's experience. In E. L. Cohen (Ed.), *Nurse case management in the 21st century* (pp. 245-255). St. Louis, MO: Mosby.

Federal Register. (1989, June 22). *Department of Education Part III: Early intervention program for infants and toddlers with handicaps: Final regulations* Vol. 54(119), 34CFR Part 303 RIN 1820-AA 49, pp. 26306-26348.

Good, M. E. (1992). The clinical nurse specialist in the school setting: Case management of migrant children with dental disease. *Clinical Nurse Specialist, 6*(2), 72-78.

Mercier, C., & Racine, G. (1995). Case management with homeless women: A descriptive study. *Community Mental Health Journal, 31*(1), 25-35.

Michaels, C. (1992). Carondelet St. Mary's nursing enterprise. *Nursing Clinics of North America, 27*(1), 77-85.

Moneyham, L., & Scott, C. B. (1997). A model emerges for the community-based nurse care management of older adults. *Nursing & Health Care Perspectives on Community, 18*(2), 68-73.

More, P. K., & Mandell, S. (1997). *Nursing case management: An evolving practice* (pp. 247-268). New York: McGraw-Hill.

Pierini, D. (1988, December). Case managing the elderly: Best bet for the future. *Health Progress, 69*(11), 42-45, 88.

Poland, M. L., Giblin, P. T., Waller, J. B., & Bayer, I. S. (1991). Development of a paraprofessional home visiting program for low-income mothers and infants. *American Journal of Preventive Medicine, 7*, 204-207.

Primomo, J. (1995). Ensuring public health nursing in managed care: partnerships for health communities. *Public Health Nursing, 12*(2), 69-71.

Resick, L. K., Taylor, C. A., Carroll, T. L., D'Antonio, J. A., & Chesnay, M. (1997). Establishing a nurse-managed wellness clinic in a predominantly older African American inner-city high rise: An advanced practice nursing project. *Nursing Administration Quarterly, 21*(4), 47-54.

Scott, J., & Rantz, M. (1997). Managing chronically ill older people in the midst of the health care revolution. *Nursing Administration Quarterly, 21*(2), 55-64.

Shamansky, S. L. (1995). A longer-than-usual editorial about population-based managed care. *Public Health Nursing, 12*(4), 211-212.

Steele, S. (1991). Nurse-case management in a rural parent-infant enrichment program. *Issues in Comprehensive Pediatric Nursing, 14*, 259-266.

Wagner, J. D., & Menke, E. M. (1992). Case management of homeless families. *Clinical Nurse Specialist, 6*(2), 65-71.

Chapter

13 Advanced Practice Nurses as Case Managers

Margaret M. Conger
Carol E. Craig

> ***CNSs have as their principal focus nursing's unique scientific and practical contributions in the management of symptoms and functional problems to meet distinctively different societal needs at the individual, group, community, and health care institution levels.***
>
> Lyon (1996)

Clinical nurse specialist (CNS), one of the roles of advanced practice nursing, requires that nurses be prepared at the master's level in nursing in a defined area of practice. CNSs' education prepares them to manage the health needs of individuals, families, and communities. They are more qualified to work with clients with complex problems because of their education in a speciality area of practice than are nurses prepared as generalists at the baccalaureate level. Clinical nurse specialists who have additional education in case management principles are particularly needed to meet the needs of the current managed care environment. Their skills are becoming recognized as important to attaining the financial and quality goals of health care organizations.

Historically, the CNS has been prepared to function in highly specialized areas within acute-care hospitals. With the rapid movement of health care into community settings, the specialized knowledge these nurses possess is now needed in community settings. Nurses with advanced education are needed to work in community settings to assist people with chronic illnesses who often have unique environmental and social conditions that place them at increased risk for health care problems. Some of them, due to poverty, lack of work-based health insurance, or chronic health problems, are not potential customers of managed care organizations. This population can best be managed by a person with case management experience.

Nurse case managers prepared at the advanced practice level are particularly skilled to intervene with clients, health care providers, and payers to promote optimum wellness (Glettler & Leen, 1996). They can assist people who have no health insurance to obtain needed health care services. In this chapter, several examples of advanced practice nurses with case management skills working in community settings will be given to demonstrate the need for nurses prepared at an advanced level of education. Included will be examples of populations with chronic illnesses such as diabetes and congestive heath failure. Populations with serious mental illness and with HIV/AIDS will also be given. Finally, the emerging field of case management with people who have sustained a work-related injury will be provided. The clinical competencies of advanced practice nursing will be applied to each of these situations. This will be followed by examples of nurses who deliver services to populations described by specific health concerns.

Advanced Practice Role: Nurse Case Manager

The introduction of nurse case managers as advanced practice nurses into community settings is a recent development; consequently this role is not well understood. The examples provided in this chapter are intended to make this role more clear. Glettler and Leen (1996) describe the advanced practice role of the nurse case manager as more complex than simply coordinating the needs of clients with payers and providers. Rather, this role is one in which the functions of interpretation, advocacy, and surveillance are superimposed over the role of coordination of services. The advanced practice nurse (APN) serves as an interpreter of information to clients and families to assist them in making informed decisions. The APN is also an advocate for the client when dealing with payers and providers of health care. A comprehensive knowledge of financial issues associated with health care payments is needed to perform this aspect of the role. In a surveillance role, the APN must constantly evaluate the outcomes of the care provided to the client and must adjust the plan of care as needed. Surveillance of use of health care dollars is also needed so that the client does not run out of benefits before the desired outcomes are met. These activities require decision-making skills best developed at the graduate level in nursing. Because the nurse case management functions described in this chapter are at an advanced practice level, the term APN will be used in the remainder of this chapter to describe this role.

The question is why an advanced practice nurse is needed to fill this role rather than a nurse with basic nursing education who also has expertise in the needs of the population served. One answer is to consider the domains of practice of the expert nursing clinician, as defined by Fenton and Brykczynski (1993) and based on the work of Benner (1984). The seven domains of advanced nursing practice are

- Diagnostic and patient monitoring
- Administering and monitoring therapeutic interventions and regimens
- Monitoring and ensuring the quality of health care practices
- Organization and work role competencies
- Helping role of the nurse
- Teaching and coaching function
- Effective management of rapidly changing situations
- Consulting role of the nurse (Fenton & Brykczynski, 1993).

The use of each of these domains will be described in reference to various populations with chronic illness served by an APN. The first example will be a population with Diabetes Mellitus Type II.

EXEMPLAR: Management of a Type II Diabetes Mellitus Population

Lisa Brugh, RN, MS

The experience of an advanced practice nurse case manager working with a population with Diabetes Mellitus Type II served through a community health center illustrates how the health of this population can be improved through education and counseling. The results of work with this population are supported by literature. A study by Coates and Boore (1996) demonstrated that provision of case management services can improve outcomes for clients with diabetes. The clients participating in their study demonstrated significant improvement in their knowledge level and self-management skills following diabetes education classes; appropriate behaviors for keeping good metabolic control, however, were rarely maintained without additional support. Coates and Boore (1996) suggest that the client must feel empowered to become an autonomous self-manager for lifestyle changes to become permanent. Ongoing education and support provided by the APN at regular intervals helped to foster such self-empowerment.

In the work described in this exemplar, the seven domains of advanced nursing practice as identified by Fenton and Brykczynski (1993) are used to illustrate the need for an advanced practice nurse.

Diagnostic and patient monitoring function. The APN works with clients with diabetes to monitor blood glucose and hemoglobin A1c levels. In addition to these chemical laboratory values that indicate a level of management of diabetes, the client's dietary habits, exercise routine, glucose monitoring and self-care functions are also monitored.

Administering and monitoring therapeutic interventions and regimens. The client's use of insulin and oral hypoglycemics is carefully followed in relationship to blood sugar levels, diet, and exercise. Recommendations to alter medication needs are made to the client's primary care provider.

Monitoring and ensuring the quality of health care practices. The APN uses clinical and functional outcomes for clients with diabetes mellitus as defined by the American Diabetic Association to assess the quality of care provided. Cost and quality outcomes are also measured.

Organizational and work-role competencies. If the client requires acute-care hospitalization, the APN must communicate with physicians, nurses, and ancillary care providers to ensure that the client's needs are met and that the overall care goals are considered. This coordination of services to maintain a continuous plan of care is necessary to maintain cost-effective care.

Helping role of the nurse. Emotional and informational support is needed by both the client and his or her family. The nurse's advocacy role is also necessary to make certain that the client is able to access the varied services required for diabetes management.

Teaching and coaching function. The provision of both individual and group teaching is a major responsibility for the APN. These activities are central to empowering clients so that they can self-manage their health status.

Effective management of rapidly changing situations. The advanced clinical skills and knowledge of the APN enable him or her to manage crises such as hypoglycemia, hyperglycemia, and acute illness experienced by clients. Facilitating access to acute-care services when needed is an important responsibility.

Consulting role of the nurse. The APN serves as an expert resource to physicians, nurses, and ancillary care providers in the care of clients with diabetes. As the person most familiar with the needs of a particular client, this role is vital to maintaining high quality services that are individualized.

Using these roles, the APN is an expert through experience and education who uses analytical and complex thought processes to manage client care. He or she relies more on deliberation and reason (rather than on intuition) in diagnosis and treatment processes than do basic practitioners (Calkin, 1984). The APN is better able to articulate the nature of nursing practice, to use reasoning to deal with practice innovations, and to develop or contribute to newer forms of practice (Calkin, 1984). Thus, the APN, as a case manager, makes an ideal person to assist the diabetic population to achieve optimal health goals.

Disease-Specific Nurse Case Management

Targeting nurse case management services to specific populations based on disease categories is on the increase for a number of reasons. To achieve the cost and quality outcomes demanded by the managed care environment, research about disease-specific management is needed. Data accumulated from large aggregates will support such a research base. A focus on a specific disease also allows the nurse to become very knowledgeable about the needs of that specific population and thus more effective in providing appropriate services. Specific diseases such as hypertension, cardiac disease, serious mental illness, diabetes mellitus, and, more recently, HIV/AIDS have been shown to use a significant percentage of available health care resources. To reduce the cost of care of these populations, effective management programs are needed. To illustrate how the use of an APN can improve care and at the same time reduce cost, examples from several of these populations will be examined.

Management of Clients With Serious Mental Illness

Nurses at the University of Cincinnati developed a walk-in psychiatric care clinic within an established "Free Store" in an inner city area (Ragiel, 1998; Ragiel, personal communication, March 1998). The clinic was funded by community mental health monies to provide counseling, medications, and case management services. The center, staffed by an APN and a social worker, began operating 4 hours a week, but the demand was so great that the hours were quickly expanded. The Health Resource Center was conceived from the beginning as an interdisciplinary practice, involving nursing, social work, and psychology. The different providers are coordinated by a nurse administrator. This model is an example of how advanced nursing practice and case management can be facilitated by an interdisciplinary team.

People with serious mental illness were provided with services such as medications, counseling, and case management for shelter and food while shopping at the Free Store for clothing and other material needs. They were also monitored for medication side effects. This walk-in clinic is an excellent example of providing care where people can easily access services and also an example of cost-effective care. The nurses demonstrated decreased emergency room visits by seriously mentally ill people in crisis, which in turn decreased costs for services, as emergency care is a very expensive means of delivering health care.

The competencies of an advanced practice nurse are needed to provide services to these clients with serious mental illness. In Table 13.1, the competencies of an advanced practice nurse (column 1) are compared to the activities of the nurse providing care to this population (column 2).

TABLE 13.1 Application of APN Competencies to Clinical Examples

APN Competency	*Seriously Mentally Ill*	*HIV/AIDS*	*CHF*[a]	*Worker's Compensation*
Diagnostic/monitoring	Monitored medication side effects	Identified social needs, monitored response to treatment modalities	Identified potential patients, monitored response to treatment modalities	Evaluated barriers to treatment
Interventions	Provided medications	Help in symptom management	Home-based care	Contacted employer for light duty, set up appointments, and accompanied client to assure information was available
Quality management		Identified and used process indicators for quality management	Monitored hospital length of stay and readmission rates	
Competencies	Interpersonal skills	Interpersonal skills	Assessment of changes in CHF status	Assessment of client and family situation; interpersonal skills
Helping role	Secured environmental needs	Assisted people to return to work without losing health benefits; linked with available services	Assisted clients and families to manage home care	Assisted client and family to manage financial, transportation, and family concerns
Teaching and coaching	Counseling	Provided education on treatment modalities, reducing possible spread of infection, and risk behavior		Education about body mechanics and personal responsibility
Consulting	Worked with inter-disciplinary team	Worked with interdisciplinary team	Consulted with home care personnel and physicians	Consulted all members of interdisciplinary team

a. CHF = congestive heart failure.

Management of Clients With HIV/AIDS

Another specific disease population positively affected by advanced practice nursing is that of people who are HIV-positive or who have AIDS. As the incidence of this disease increases across the country, demands for services are straining the resources of every health care organization. Although new breakthroughs in medical treatment have extended the lives and the quality of life for many people with AIDS, every successful effort to manage this population in a community setting rather than within the acute-care hospital is important. The specific needs of this population require that coordinated efforts by health care providers knowledgeable about disease management and health promotion be available.

Needs specific to this population arise throughout the course of the disease. At the point of diagnosis, clients need both education on how to diminish the spread of the disease to unaffected contacts and encouragement to reduce risk-taking activities. The client also needs education at this point about treatment modalities that will slow the course of the disease. Medications to reduce viral load are extremely expensive, and many people will need assistance in finding funding sources. The use of protease inhibitors has resulted in dramatic improvements in slowing or stopping disease progression in many people who were extremely ill. For those who are benefitting from new drugs, the challenge has become learning to live, rather than preparing for death (Sowell, 1997). Assisting people to return to work without losing health care benefits has become a new challenge for advanced nurse practitioners who work with the HIV-infected population (Sowell, 1997). As the disease progresses through a series of opportunistic infections, the need for help in managing the treatment modalities increases. And finally, as the client approaches the terminal phase of the disease, the need for case management increases to help meet the social and emotional issues, as well as the physical problems.

Nurses who have been educated to work with this specific population are more effective than those who have had only limited contact with HIV/AIDS clients, due to the specific treatment required for the management of this disease (Sowell, 1997). Clients with HIV/AIDS tend to be very knowledgeable about their disease, often knowing more about the latest research findings than the average health care provider. To maintain credibility with these clients, the nurse must spend considerable time staying abreast of the latest findings.

The need for assistance in finding adequate medical care and social service supports needed by these clients can be overwhelming. Sowell (1995) identified social needs of this group as including housing arrangements, food resources, transportation assistance, and treatment for drug and alcohol addiction. Some of these problems are related to the increase in incidence of disease among people who are homeless or suffering from chronic mental illness.

The goal of a program for the HIV/AIDS population is to maximize each person's functional status and promote well-being (Sowell, 1995). One of the greatest needs is to link each individual with appropriate services. In the short perspective, such actions may appear to increase total costs; in the long term, such actions will reduce the need for more expensive health care services. To be able to effectively carry out these needed activities, the competencies of the APN are needed. Again, a comparison of the APN's competencies with the activities needed to manage clients with HIV/AIDS is shown in Table 13.1.

Some research studies show that nurse case management of clients with HIV/AIDS can have a positive effect on the person's function and reduce cost (Nickel et al., 1996). It has been difficult, however, to measure positive outcomes from such programs with this group because of the progressive nature of the disease. Classical outcome indicators such as mortality or morbidity are not very useful. Evaluation based on process indicators such as the number of persons served, a decrease in the number of acute-care hospital days to manage the opportunistic infections, and, most important, the number of people educated about means to prevent spread of the infection may be the most appropriate way to evaluate the effect of nurse case management in this population (Sowell, 1995).

Management of Clients With Congestive Heart Failure

Case management services are also needed that move across boundaries of community- and hospital-based care. With a number of chronic diseases, there is a need to manage clients so that the community-based care coordinates well with the hospital-based nursing staff. An example of how such coordination can enhance the well-being of clients with congestive heart failure while reducing health care costs is provided by Donlevy and Pietruch (1996). The nursing staff at the Good Samaritan Hospital in Lebanon, Pennsylvania identified patients with the medical diagnosis of congestive heart failure

(CHF) as at high risk for frequent readmission. CHF patients were commonly readmitted within 15 days of discharge with exacerbations of their condition. In an effort to reduce the cost of health care, this population was targeted for a special program using community-based case managers. The hospital staff nurses were cross-trained in home health nursing concepts and worked in conjunction with experienced home health nurses in delivering home-based care to this population.

A home-care clinical pathway for the CHF patient, specific educational tools, and a screening tool to identify potential persons needing this service were developed by the APN. Criteria for inclusion in the program included one or more of the following: a new diagnosis of CHF, readmission with CHF within 31 days, taking five or more cardiac drugs, identified need for teaching about the disease and its management, or a pattern of noncompliance with treatment regimen (Donlevy & Pietruch, 1996). In addition to case management while in the hospital, each client received a telephone call shortly after discharge, and home-care visits were provided as needed. These interventions are compared with the competencies of an APN and shown in Table 13.1.

The outcomes achieved by this program have been significant. Only two clients were readmitted to the hospital within 31 days for problems with management of CHF following initiation of the program. For those who were readmitted at a later time, the average length of stay (LOS) was 3.5 days, compared to an average LOS of 8.6 days prior to the beginning of this program, thus reducing the cost of hospital care. This program is an excellent example of how population-based case management targeted at a client group with a history of expensive health care costs can be used to better achieve desired cost-effectiveness needed by managed care organizations.

EXEMPLAR: Worker's Compensation-Based Case Management

Deanne Lewis, RN, MS, and Teri Fernandez, RN, MS

Another area in which nurses are developing community-based case management programs is worker's compensation programs. These claims sometimes arise out of injuries that are very extensive or that could lead to a chronic problem; at other times, the injury many lead to a situation in which fragmentation of medical care has occurred. When an insurance company is faced with an complex claim arising out of a work-related injury, it is the goal of both the insurance company and the injured worker to provide services that will result in a safe return to work in a timely manner. In a worker's compensation case, the insurer must pay both the medical expenses and at least a part of lost wages (Mullahy, 1995). Thus the interest of the insurer is to promote the employee to return to work as quickly as possible. To achieve this goal, the insurance company will often contract with a case management company to handle complex cases that could be very costly to the insurance company.

Management of worker's compensation cases is a growing area of entrepreneurship for APNs. When the APN receives a referral from the insurance provider, a comprehensive assessment of the client and his or her home environment will be conducted. Mullahy (1995) recommends that this assessment be conducted in the client's home because the home dynamics may present unforeseen management problems. The APN will need to use prudence in determining if there are possible safety issues for the nurse that could preclude conducting the interview in the home. This assessment will include a review of financial, health, psychosocial, and environmental issues. Using the data obtained from this assessment, the nurse will then develop a plan of care for the client in collaboration with the client's physician. Together the APN and the physician will present the recommendations for treatment management to the insurance company. When the treatment plan is approved by all parties, the APN will collaborate with all of the care providers, such as physical therapists, occupational therapists, or respiratory therapists, to ensure continuity, progress, and quality of care. The nurse will keep the client informed of needed appointments with physicians and other health care providers, make certain that all of the information needed is available at the appointment, and follow up with the client to ensure that follow-up care is done. The APN often attends many of the appointments with the client to facilitate understanding and communication. He or she also keeps in contact with all physicians involved in the client's care so that the treatment plan moves forward as agreed.

The insurance provider benefits from this service by reducing redundancy in care and ensuring that all services are provided in a timely manner. This coordination of care leads to reduced costs because each encounter of the client and health care provider is focused on meeting the primary need. Time is not lost in misunderstanding of the treatment plan. The insurance provider benefits in that the APN prevents services from "falling though the cracks," leading to lost time and effort. The client benefits because the APN acts as the client's advocate in obtaining services, enhancing recovery. Having a nurse present to answer the client's questions, interpret physician reports, and cut through bureaucratic problems makes for a satisfied customer. Such satisfaction is important to the insurance company because a happy client will be more cooperative with the program and will not seek legal representation.

The following example is an actual case of a worker's compensation claim that occurred without the benefit of case management services. Following this example is a scenario of how this case could have been managed by an APN. The cost differences are explored illustrating the financial advantages of using an APN with clients who have potentially troubling compensation claims.

TL is a 42-year-old male employed by a sheet-metal manufacturing company. After returning from lunch one day, TL was lifting a stack of sheet metal, estimated to weigh about 40 lb, over his head. During the lift, he suddenly experienced a sharp pain in his mid-lower back. He described this pain as a popping sensation. He reported the injury immediately to his supervisor and a coworker drove him to an Urgent Care Center (UCC).

The attending UCC physician examined him and ordered that some X rays of his back be taken. The initial reading from these X rays indicated moderate degenerative changes, nonspecific in nature. The diagnosis given was lower back pain and sprain/strain syndrome. TL was sent home with a prescription for a nonsteroidal anti-inflammatory drug (NSAID) and an over-the-counter pain medication. He was told to stay home from work for 1 week and to follow up with his primary care physician. TL informed his employer of the physician order to stay home from work but did not start taking the NSAID prescription for 3 days. He did take some ibuprofen that he had in his medicine cabinet.

Week 1 of Claim

TL followed up with a visit to his primary care physician and reported, "I feel a little better and I only took a few NSAID pills, I didn't know that it was important. They bother my stomach." His physician encouraged him to take the NSAID and the ibuprofen, remain off work, and start physical therapy 3 days a week. At the time of the visit, the X ray taken at the time of injury was not available to the physician. A request was sent to the UCC to obtain the X ray so that the physician could review it when TL returned for a follow-up visit in 2 weeks.

The physical therapy referral was never initiated because TL waited to be called to be told when to start his appointments. During the next 2 weeks, TL's condition regressed, with an increase in his lower back pain and additional pains shooting down both legs. He slept on the couch at night because he found his bed uncomfortable. During the day, he cared for his 2-year-old son while his wife was working at a temporary job to "make ends meet."

Week 3

At the next appointment with the physician, an MRI was ordered and the plan for physical therapy was put on hold until the results of the MRI were obtained. TL was told to return to follow up with the physician in 1 week. Three days after this appointment, the report from the MRI was obtained, revealing moderate bulges at lumbars 3, 4, and 5 and sacral 1 vertebrae.

Week 4

TL missed his next scheduled appointment with his physician. No action was taken at this time.

Week 5

At this time, TL received a phone call from the Worker's Compensation claims manager, who wanted to know about his medical status and his return-to-work status. This phone call encouraged TL to make an appointment with his physician, and he was able to schedule a visit in 3 days. At this visit, he was given the results found on the MRI and was advised to continue with his physical therapy treatments. TL informed the physician that he had never started the treatments. He was told to start the physical therapy program and return to see the physician in 2 weeks. TL did start the physical therapy three times a week for 2 weeks. During that time, he worked with several different therapists and missed two appointments.

Week 7

At TL's next physician appointment, the physical therapy evaluations were not available for review, but TL reported that his pain was now contained to his lower back area. He still was having difficulty sleeping, felt very stressed, and had frequent headaches. The physician prescribed continuing the physical therapy treatments, changed the medication to Flexeril and Paxil, and asked that TL return for follow-up in 2 weeks.

Week 13

The pattern described above continued another 6 weeks with no improvement in TL's condition. He reported that he had started drinking several beers at night to help him sleep. His pain continued, he was depressed and angry, and he was unable to return to work. His financial status was causing him great concern; his wife took a full-time job, receiving minimum wage. The family was in near-crisis status, and a brother-in-law encouraged TL to seek an attorney to represent him in a suit against his company.

Alternate Scenario, With APN-Nurse Case Manager Involvement

The following example describes how an APN would have managed this situation. The benefits derived from such management will become apparent.

Week 4

The employer's insurance company identified that this claim was becoming problematic and made contact with an APN to investigate the claim. The APN would call TL and make an appointment for an initial evaluation. During this evaluation, the APN could establish a trusting relationship with TL and identify the following barriers to care:

- Transportation: TL has a five-speed 1983 4-wheel-drive vehicle that causes him pain when he gets in and out and when he tries to shift. Thus TL is unable to drive himself to his health care appointments.
- Body mechanics: judged to be poor. TL is frequently seen bending over to lift his 32-pound son.
- Understanding of responsibility: judged to lack a clear understanding of his responsibility to communicate with his employer concerning his off-work status.
- Financial concerns: judged to be acute, leading to considerable stress.

Interventions. The APN would contact TL's employer and discuss the possibility of finding a "light duty" position. She would discuss with them the benefits that a light duty position would provide; namely, helping the employee maintain work pattern behaviors that could increase the speed of recovery. The APN also would communicate with all health care providers, obtain all records, and facilitate an appointment with the physician.

Week 5

The APN would accompany TL to the next physician visit, making sure that all physical therapy and X-ray reports were available to the physician. During the next few weeks, the APN would provide TL with emotional support, therapeutic communication, and education about the treatment regimen. During that time she would monitor TL's body mechanics to ensure that he was following the physical therapist's instructions. TL would be able to return to work in a light duty position, using a car pool arrangement, and the family financial strain would be reduced. The APN would also make arrangements for transportation for TL to get to all medical appointments. Over this period, TL will retain his self-esteem and feel supported by his health care team and his employer.

Week 9

The outcome of these interventions would be that TL will return to his usual and customary job with no residual impairments from his injury. Furthermore, there will be no discussion of obtaining an attorney. The interventions provided are compared with APN competencies as described by Fenton and Brykczynski (1993) and are shown in Table 13.1. Care provided by an APN can result in an increased quality of life for TL as well achieving cost benefits for the insurance provider.

The cost benefits of using an APN to coordinate TL's treatment plan are enormous. Table 13.2 provides an analysis of costs for the management of TL with and without nurse case management involvement. The total cost savings achieved when the case was coordinated by the APN was $46,305. A very significant difference was the amount of wages lost to TL. Without case management, TL was out of work for 6 months, with a loss of $14,400. With case management, he lost only 6 weeks of work. TL required nine visits with a physician without case management; this was reduced to four visits with

TABLE 13.2 Comparison of Worker's Compensation Costs

	Without Case Management	*With Case Management*
Lost wages	$14,400	$ 3,600
MD charges	755	410
Medications	425	25
Physical therapy	6,840	1,080
Insurance attorney	20,000	0
Nurse case manager	0	1,000
Total costs	$52,420	$6,115
Net savings with case management		$46,305

case management. The difference in the cost of physical therapy was also significant. Without case management, this would come to $6,840; with case management it was reduced to $1,080. Even the difference in cost of medication was significant, with a cost of $425 without case management and only $25 with case management. The cost without the coordination of the APN was considerably increased because of TL's decision to use an attorney to handle his case because of dissatisfaction with his medical management. The attorney charges that had to be paid by the insurance company came to $20,000. This case illustrates that coordination of services by an APN can provide both increased quality of care to the client and considerable cost savings to the insurance company.

Conclusions

Advanced practice nurses are aware of the health care needs of populations at risk and know how to develop programs that are specific to these needs. The providers working with this group can become expert in developing effective interventions. Because many of these subpopulations have been shown to use health care resources inefficiently, programs that improve health practices can have a significant impact on the cost of health care. In an era of scarce resources, such efforts are worth pursuing.

Nurses have demonstrated that population-based health care is an area that deserves increased attention. New educational programs need to be developed to prepare nurses for this practice. First, a strong grounding in public health principles is needed for the nurse to be successful, along with the development of excellent collaborative skills so he or she can work effectively in team settings. This is a practice area for nurses prepared at the graduate level who have developed the independent nursing skills needed to function in the community in an autonomous practice.

References

Benner, P. (1984). *From novice to expert.* Menlo Park, CA: Addison Wesley.

Calkin, J. D. (1984). A model for advanced nursing practice. *Journal of Nursing Administration, 14*(1), 24-30.

Coates, V. E., & Boore, J.R.P. (1996). Knowledge and diabetes self-management. *Patient Education and Counseling, 29*(1), 99-108.

Donlevy, J. A., & Pietruch, B. L. (1996). The connection delivery model: Care across the continuum. *Nursing Management, 27*(5), 34, 36.

Fenton, M., & Brykczynski, K. A. (1993). Qualitative distinctions and similarities in the practice of clinical nurse specialists and nurse practitioners. *Journal of Professional Nursing, 9*(6), 313-326.

Glettler, E., & Leen, M. G. (1996). The advanced practice nurse as case manager. *Journal of Case Management, 5*(3), 121-126.

Lyon, B. L. (1996, June 15). Meeting societal needs for CNS competencies: Why the CNS and NP roles should not be blended in masters degree programs. Retrieved September 4, 1998, from the World Wide Web: http://www.nursingworld.org/ojin

Mullahy, C. M. (1995). *The case manager's handbook.* Gaithersburg, MD: Aspen.

Nickel, J. T., Salsberry, P. J., Caswell, R. J., Keller, M. D., Long, T., & O'Connell, M. (1996). Quality of life in nurse case management of persons with AIDS receiving home care. *Research in Nursing & Health, 19*(92), 91-99.

Ragiel, E. (1998, February). *Management of clients with serious mental illness.* Paper presented at the American Association of Clinical Nurses Faculty Practice Conference, Phoenix, AZ.

Sowell, J. (1995, January 9). HIV/AIDS prevention knowledge and behaviors among persons seeking services at an HIV organization. *AIDS Weekly*, 27.

Sowell, J. (1997). AIDS care reconstruction. *Journal of the Association of Nurses in AIDS Care, 8*(6), 43-46.

Chapter

14

Advanced Practice Roles in Community Settings

Community Health Clinics

Carol E. Craig
Kathy Ingleses
Margaret M. Conger

> ***Nursing has always responded to society's health care needs. Whether this response has been to care for soldiers to meet their needs, as Florence Nightingale did, or to bring health care to the community as Lillian Wald did . . . nurses have engaged in expanded roles.***
>
> **O'Flynn (1996)**

Advanced practice nurses (APNs) have a long history of commitment to deliver health care to populations that fall outside of mainstream health services. These services can be provision of direct primary health care delivered by a nurse practitioner, or they may be case management services provided by an APN case manager. The nature of the service is directed by the needs of the population. Establishment of primary health care centers that provide health promotion and disease prevention services as well as diagnosis and management of illness is a developing strategy. Clients using health centers sometimes require services beyond those the center can offer. An important service that nurses offer is to link the client with services in the larger community.

There are many reasons why a specific population may choose to use a community health center rather than a mainstream health service. Often the choice is based on access. For example, teenagers may not have access to common health services due to lack of transportation or due to a lack of trust in health care providers associated with mainstream services. Another group that falls outside mainstream health services is the medically uninsured. Uninsured people often have access to medical services only in crisis situations. Sometimes people are unable to access care because they are homeless or are migrant workers. Others without health care are the working poor, who are in more stable living situations but do not have discretionary income to afford health services.

To serve the needs of disenfranchised populations, APNs have developed health centers in proximity to populations in need. In the development of a successful community center, the APN usually incorporates the help of community members to aid residents in understanding that the center is their own place. This encourages an atmosphere of acceptance, where people are comfortable to discuss health concerns. In this chapter, the needs of underserved populations and health centers that service their needs will be explored.

Health Management: The Teen Population

Adolescents in the United States are generally thought to be a healthy population (Kisker & Brown, 1996). Adolescent health is assumed to be good in the United States because we live in a country that enjoys one of the highest standards of living in the world (Miller, 1990). It is true that adolescents benefit from low rates of mortality, disease-related morbidity, or disability associated with disease (Holden & Nitz, 1995), but they are experiencing increased health risks due to social, economic, and behavioral factors (Siegel, 1995).

These "social morbidities" result from lifestyle practices that include, but are not limited to, substance use and abuse, violence, suicide, teen pregnancy, sexually transmitted diseases, and eating disorders (DiClemente, Hansen, & Ponton, 1996). Although preventable aspects of morbidity and mortality related to behavioral risk-taking behaviors are important, assessment of risk-taking behaviors over the long term is also necessary. What will happen to these adolescents as they enter adulthood? Social and psychological indicators such as well-being, education and job performance, quality of family and social relations, and future economic stability are also at stake for adolescents who take risks (DiClemente et al., 1996).

Unfortunately, health outcomes for adolescents engaging in risk-taking behaviors are becoming more problematic (DiClemente et al., 1996). First, initiation of risk-taking behavior is occurring at younger ages. Second, the number of adolescents who live in poverty is increasing, and poor youth face a greater risk of impaired physical and psychological health (DiClemente et al., 1996). These trends suggest that more young people will be vulnerable to experimentation that not only has harmful health effects during adolescence but may also result in health consequences for them in the future (Hedberg, Byrd, Klein, Auinger, & Weitzman, 1996).

A growing segment of the adolescent population is uninsured or underinsured for health care (DiClemente et al., 1996). Lack of insurance produces obstacles ranging from limited access to services, lack of resources, and lack of transportation to get to where low-cost services are (Kisker & Brown, 1996). Clearly, adolescents have many health needs, yet often few resources are available to address those needs.

Models of Care for Adolescents

Several innovative models of care address the unique needs of adolescents. A traditional model is the community health center. A newer, more focused model of a community health center is the school-based, school-linked clinic. Regardless of the model of service, essential components of adolescent health care programs must include a comprehensive package of prevention, education, and physical and mental health services (Hedberg et al., 1996; Kisker & Brown, 1996; Miller, 1996; U.S. Congress, 1991).

Traditional Community Health Center-Based Care for Adolescents

Hedberg et al. (1996) analyzed data from the 1988 National Health Interview Survey and looked at a sample of 6,635 adolescents from 11 to 17 years old. Community health centers (CHCs) were an important source of preventive care for impoverished adolescents. Adolescents who used the CHCs had greater psychosocial problems but used the CHC as regularly as those who used family practice settings. CHCs were used for primary care services; therefore periodic comprehensive visits to CHCs may be an effective way to deliver preventive health care to adolescents. Unfortunately, little information is available about preventive education provided during an adolescent's visit to a CHC, and it is not known if improved health outcomes resulted from preventive information (Hedberg et al., 1996).

School-Based, School-Linked Community Health Centers

Affecting health outcomes through the provision of school-based clinics or in collaboration with schools is promising (Kisker & Brown, 1996; Miller, 1990). Kisker and Brown (1996) analyzed 24 school-based health centers (SBHCs), all of which received Robert Wood Johnson Foundation monies to initiate school-based clinics. The clinics were in a variety of settings: schools, public health departments, hospitals, and nonprofit institutions. The health centers were awarded monies based on their service to secondary school students with substantial unmet health care needs. Two objectives for the foundation grant were to determine if the centers (a) increased access to basic health care services and (b) reduced the prevalence of high-risk behaviors, including substance use and unprotected sexual activity. Kisker and Brown found that school-based health centers increased students' access to health care and improved their health knowledge. No significant data, however, demonstrated a reduction in high-risk behaviors (Kisker & Brown, 1996).

Clinical Example

A school-linked clinic shown to be successful in improving adolescent health is The Teen Clinic (Teen Wellness Center) in Flagstaff, Arizona (Coconino County Department of Health Services, 1998). The clinic was originally established in 1990 as a result of a Flagstaff Youth Town Hall meeting where youth of the town expressed their desire for free, confidential health care services. The Coconino County Department of Health Services and The Guidance Center (a behavioral/mental health facility) collaborated in starting the clinic to provide pregnancy testing and counseling. Services quickly expanded to provide primary health care for people 13 to 19 years old, including physical, behavioral, mental health, and social services.

The Teen Clinic is open three afternoons a week on a first-come, first-served, walk-in basis. An appointment system was used initially, but the majority of teens did not return for their appointments. A fourth day may be added to the clinic schedule to accommodate appointments for follow-up issues. The clinic is nurse managed, and the staff comprises two nurses, a nurse practitioner, and a social and behavioral health worker. Because the nurse practitioner's time and the behavioral health specialist's time are limited to clinic hours only, the nurses are the case managers. The two baccalaureate-prepared nurses are responsible for clinic flow. The RN role is to assess all clients, address client questions and problems, and then to triage clients to the appropriate member of the team. The RN assessment includes not only physical and psychological health issues but assessment and referral to other community resources. The nurses educate and counsel on both wellness and illness issues, including birth control methods, STD prevention, signs and symptoms of illness, and medication regimens. They provide referrals for more complex health problems, dental issues, and complex medical and behavioral health. Any problems that may be beyond the RN scope of practice are discussed with the nurse practitioner and/or the behavioral health specialist.

The nurse practitioner assesses and diagnoses wellness and illness concerns, performs physical exams, prescribes and dispenses medications, and makes referrals as necessary. The behavioral health specialist is responsible for pregnancy testing and counseling and also addresses such issues as decision making, responsibility and choice, rape, family violence, suicide, and substance abuse. The nurses then manage follow-up based on the nurse practitioner's or the behavioral health specialist's plan, including follow-up with parents as necessary and communication with school nurses. This is a team approach, and each member is an integral part in working to provide the best care for adolescents.

In 1997, over 2,000 adolescents and their families were seen in The Teen Clinic for a variety of primary care issues. When the clinic first started, 75%

of the clients were seen for pregnancy testing and family planning. Currently 50% of the visits address behavioral and mental health issues. One positive health outcome is the reduction in the teen pregnancy rate. When the Teen Wellness Center was initiated in 1990, the teen pregnancy rate for Coconino County was 8% and the city of Flagstaff's rate was 7%. As of December 1997, the Coconino County Teen pregnancy rate is 4.25% and the city of Flagstaff's rate is 3% (Coconino County Department of Health Services, 1998).

In summary, adolescents face many problems. Teens are generally healthy, but many of their health problems revolve around risk-taking behaviors. Several models of delivery and provision of health care to adolescents were shown to increase access to services and to increase awareness of potential health-related risk factors. Innovative programs will, it is hoped, show positive effects on health outcomes.

Health Management: Uninsured Populations

Nurse-managed health centers have been established to serve the needs of the "notch group": those who make a modest salary and are above the income levels for government-sponsored health insurance but who do not have employer-sponsored health care.

One such project is the North Country Community Health Center (NCCHC) in Flagstaff, Arizona. The NCCHC began as a community partnership with concerned Flagstaff citizens and nursing faculty members at Northern Arizona University (Craig, 1996). Clients using this health center are primarily the working poor, with few resources and little or no discretionary income. People who come to the health center often have long-standing health concerns. Known health problems may go untreated due to an inability to afford either treatment or the medication to manage chronic problems. Many in this population speak only Spanish, compounding their difficulty in getting appropriate care.

Nurse practitioners working at the health center take responsibility for managing the diagnosis and treatment of chronic and acute health problems. They work alongside nurse case managers who are involved in education programs regarding chronic illness and in working with clients to obtain needed community services. Common health problems are obesity associated with either (or, often, both) diabetes mellitus or hypertension. At times, medical services that are beyond the scope of the health center are identified.

When this occurs, the APNs must work with existing acute-care providers in the community to obtain needed care.

One of the programs offered at the health center is case management that focuses on assisting clients with dietary and exercise lifestyle changes. Education about chronic illness and strategies to improve health are also included. Strategies culturally appropriate for this population were developed that have proven to be effective. Many of the clients were able to reduce their weight over a 3-month period by improving their dietary habits and increasing or beginning a moderate exercise program. Changes in lifestyle habits resulted in a lowering of blood sugar and blood pressure. With collaboration of nurse practitioners and nurse case managers, many clients with chronic health problems reduced the need for acute hospitalization.

To demonstrate the types of nursing interventions used with these clients, records were maintained using the Nursing Intervention Classification system (McCloskey & Bulechek, 1996). This system provides a comprehensive classification of the types of treatments performed by nurses and can be used to standardize descriptions of what nurses do when working with clients. With the use of this classification, all nurses working in case management will record their interventions using a standard language. Such standardization leads to better communication among providers and also improves continuity of client care (McCloskey & Bulechek, 1996). Another advantage of this system is that each intervention has a code number that can be input into a computer database. With this capability of computerization, it is possible to retrieve actual data about what nurses do. The following clinical example demonstrates the effectiveness of such services.

Clinical Example

Molly was a woman in her 60s who came to the health center for medication to manage her high blood pressure and diabetes. She last saw a physician almost 8 months before, when she lost her job and her insurance. She had been out of medication for about 6 weeks when she heard about the health center. She stated that she felt well but was concerned about her medications. On examination, she was found to have diabetic neuropathy in her feet, 4+ protein in her urine, hemoglobin A1c of 7.2, a cardiac risk ratio of 9.6, and a blood pressure of 152/110. She had little knowledge about either

her hypertension or her diabetes. She was referred to the nurse case manager for education about both conditions.

During the initial case management interview, Molly talked about her inability to exercise due to pain in her right hip. She had difficulty with weight bearing and walked with severe pain. Her pain prevented her from participating in an exercise program needed to promote weight reduction. Molly had extensive teaching about a low-fat, diabetic diet. She started on medications, including a lipid-lowering drug. She was also provided with a blood glucose monitoring device and taught how to use it.

After a year in case management, she had lowered her cardiac risk to 7.9 and her hemoglobin A1c to 6.4. During this time, she began to have chest pain, shortness of breath, and swollen ankles and was diagnosed with congestive heart failure. Molly was referred to a cardiologist by the family nurse practitioner (FNP), who offered his services to the health center once a month. He recommended that she have a stress EKG as soon as possible. She lived with her two daughters and three grandchildren on a very limited income. No money was available either for the test or for any subsequent surgery. She was several years away from Medicare eligibility and was a few dollars over the qualifying income for state Medicaid help.

The nurse case manager went with the patient to the Medicaid office to discuss what Molly would need to do to qualify for assistance. If Molly incurred just a few hundred dollars more in medical bills, she would be eligible. The NCM subsequently approached the local hospital administrator, where the stress EKG would be done, to request that Molly be allowed to have the test without prior payment. The request was granted. The findings of the stress EKG indicated a need for a coronary catheterization. Again, the hospital administrator was approached for permission to go ahead with the test prior to determining the payment source. It was obvious to both the nurse case manager and the hospital financial advisor that the cost of these two tests would be sufficient to qualify Molly for the state Medicaid program. In Arizona, the Medicaid program will pay medical bills that are incurred just before the patient becomes eligible for assistance. The hospital agreed to have Molly undergo the cardiac catheterization, and the cardiologist who had seen her at the health center waived his fee for performing the test. The NCM worked with Molly to help her make a decision about going forward with the test and helped prepare her for it. As a result of all this expensive testing, Molly became eligible to receive health care for 6 months under the Medicaid program.

Subsequent to the cardiac catheterization, Molly was referred to another hospital for an angioplasty procedure to improve the circulation through her coronary arteries. This, of course, was covered by the state health plan. While she was covered by insurance, the NCM encouraged Molly to have a hip repair also, to reduce her hip pain. She qualified for the replacement, which was done 5 months after her angioplasty.

Unfortunately, while Molly was on the Medicaid program, she was followed in a traditional medical model by her specialists. She no longer received services at the Health Center and was lost from the nurse case manager's caseload. Without the encouragement that the NCM provided, Molly's clinical status deteriorated. She returned to the Health Center for care 1 year later when she no longer qualified for Medicare funding. At that time, her hemoglobin A1c had risen to 7.9 and her cardiac risk was 11.0. She had significantly increased the diabetic neuropathy in her feet and was not following her prescribed diet. The FNP and NCM concluded that her angioplasty and hip replacement were far less effective than anticipated because she was unable to control the underlying causes of her condition. Molly's need for intensive case management services to help her regain self-care management was recognized and a referral was made to the case manager.

During the period of case management, a number of nursing interventions were used. These are described using the Nursing Interventions Classification (NIC) terminology and are shown are shown in Table 14.1. They are organized using the domains established by McCloskey and Bulechek (1996). Interventions from the physiological domains, both basic and complex, were used. Interventions from the behavior and health system domains were also used. The interventions used demonstrate the holistic approach to care that can be managed by advanced practice nurses.

This example demonstrates how health care can be provided in a manner that improves self-management skills and at the same time allows for quality services. The future of health care needs to move in this direction. Nurses can demonstrate a significant impact on reducing health care costs through the use of APNs in community settings.

Conclusions

This chapter provides several examples of APN practice that meet the challenges of populations that fall outside the mainstream of health delivery

TABLE 14.1 Nursing Interventions Used With Client

Physiological: basic	
Activity and exercise management	
0200	Exercise promotion
Nutrition support	
5246	Nutritional counseling
1280	Weight reduction assistance
Physiological: complex	
Drug management	
5616	Teaching prescribed medications
Behavioral	
Coping assistance	
5250	Decision-making support
Patient education	
5510	Health education
Health system	
Health system mediation	
7400	Health system guidance
2880	Preoperative coordination
Health system management	
7610	Bedside laboratory testing
Information management	
7960	Health care information exchange
8020	Multidisciplinary care conference

services. The success of services for populations at risk is demonstrated when expensive acute-care services are reduced by early detection and management of chronic problems. Quality of care is also important to increase quality of life.

Advanced practice nurses demonstrated that they are both cost efficient and deliver quality care to underserved populations. The practices described in this chapter should be expanded to meet larger numbers of people who fall outside of the health care delivery system. In the next chapter, a collaborative model using advanced practice nurses will be explored in more depth.

References

Coconino County Department of Health Services. (1998). *Community based services: School based, school-linked services* (Quarterly report). Flagstaff, AZ: Author.

Craig, C. (1996). Making the most of a nurse-managed clinic. *Nursing and Health Care, 17*(3), 124-126.

DiClemente, R. J., Hansen, W. B., & Ponton, L. E. (1996). Adolescents at risk. In R. J. DiClemente, W. B. Hansen, & L. E. Ponton (Eds.), *Handbook of adolescent health risk behavior* (pp. 1-4). New York: Plenum.

Hedberg, V. A., Byrd, R. S., Klein, J. D., Auinger, P., & Weitzman, M. (1996). The role of community health centers in providing preventive care to adolescents. *Archives of Pediatric and Adolescent Medicine, 150,* 603-608.

Holden, E. W., & Nitz, K. (1995). Epidemiology of adolescent health disorders. In J. L. Wallander & L. J. Siegel (Eds.), *Adolescent health problems: Behavioral perspectives* (pp. 7-21). New York: Guilford.

Kisker, E. E., & Brown, R. S. (1996). Do school-based health centers improve adolescents' access to health care, health status, and risk-taking behavior? *Journal of Adolescent Health, 18,* 335-343.

Miller, D. F. (1990). *The case for school-based health clinics.* Bloomington, IN: Phi Delta Kappa Educational Foundation.

McCloskey, J. C., & Bulechek, G. M. (1996). *Nursing intervention classification.* St. Louis, MO: Mosby.

O'Flynn, A. L. (1996). The preparation of advanced practice nurses. *Nursing Clinics of North America, 31*(3), 429-437.

Siegel, L. J. (1995). Overview. In J. L. Wallander & L. J. Siegel (Eds.), *Adolescent health problems: Behavioral perspectives* (pp. 3-6). New York: Guilford.

U.S. Congress, Office of Technology Assessment. (1991). *Adolescent health. Vol. 3. Cross-cutting issues in the delivery of health and related services* (Pub. No. OTA-H-467). Washington, DC: U.S. Government Printing Office.

Chapter

15

Advanced Nurse Collaborative Practice in a Primary Care Setting

Carol E. Craig
Margaret M. Conger

Well now, if you walk up and down with your umbrella, saying "Tut-tut, it looks like rain," I shall do what I can by singing a little Cloud Song, such as a cloud might sing.
Winnie the Pooh **(A. A. Milne)**

Just as Winnie the Pooh needed the help of Christopher Robin to achieve his goal of reaching the honey in the tree, health care providers need the help of each other to achieve their goals in working with clients in need of health care. Collaboration with one another is often the key to achieving one's goal. Pooh had tried to reach the honey on his own, but met with an unfortunate fall into a gorse bush. It was only when he thought of Christopher Robin as a potential colleague in his effort that he was able to work out a plan to reach the honey.

Both Pooh and Christopher Robin had separate and distinct abilities. Pooh's ability was to be a rain cloud, so that the bees would not become suspicious. Christopher Robin's ability was to distract the bees by pretending he saw a rain cloud up near the tree instead of a "silly old bear." But together they were able to carry out the plan. In the same way, advanced practice nurses (APNs) can work together to assist their clients to achieve their goals. This chapter will explore how two distinct and separate APN practices, that of a family nurse practitioner (FNP) and of a nurse case manager (NCM), can work together, each using their own distinct skills. Such collaboration is a model that needs to be encouraged.

Need for APNs in Primary Health Care Settings

Nurses frequently work with clients in primary care settings who have little or limited health care. Populations with underserved health needs include people who are often at the greatest risk for health problems, including those with multiple health care concerns and limited environmental and social resources. Providing high-quality, cost-effective primary care for a high-risk population is difficult when a medical model is used, due to the complexity of the social and environmental problems that these people face. At this time, most primary health centers within the managed care environment rely on medical model approaches. People presenting with multiple complex social and health needs, however, require a more holistic approach.

Populations with complex needs present a challenge to health care systems that could be met with the use of APNs, for APNs have the appropriate education to assess and manage complex health care needs in a holistic manner and to understand the importance of environmental, social, and cultural influences on health. Different types of advanced practice nurses, working in partnership in new roles and relationships, can provide the backbone of primary care (Walker & Sebastian, 1997), especially within a community-based system. A partnership between FNPs and NCMs in primary care is a new model for care. Pender (1992) believed that partnership was a viable alternative to "rugged individualism" in health care. Haddock (1997) states that NCMs focus on collaboration and consultation *between* disciplines. Consultation and collaboration *within* the discipline of nursing is a new concept that can provide high-quality, cost-effective care. This chapter will describe the changing roles of advanced practice nurses, present a model of collaborative nursing practice for APNs, and describe the partnership between an FNP and a nurse case manager in a community health center as an illustration of the possibilities for new partnerships.

Evolving Roles for Advanced Practice Nurses

Changes in advanced nursing practice are reflected in the nursing literature by debates on education and appropriate roles and tasks for APNs. Historically, nurses who practiced beyond the basic level included clinical nurse specialists (CNSs), nurse practitioners (NPs), nurse midwives, and nurse anesthetists. With the advent of managed care, case management became a new field for advanced practice nurses, although not all case managers are prepared at the master's level or are nurses (Jenkins & Sullivan-Marx, 1994). Many NCMs have evolved from clinical nurse specialists who changed their focus. The case manager role has been called by some nurses the "third generation" of CNSs (Haddock, 1997). CNSs are developing case management skills in response to a changing health care environment and to new opportunities for advanced nursing practice (Haddock, 1997).

Some nurses advocate for an APN who is educated and capable of managing both NP and CNS functions. The argument is that advanced practice roles are merging, and CNSs and NPs will be doing the same functions in the future (Elder & Bullough, 1990; Schroer, 1991). Cronenwett (1995) stated that combining roles and titles will reduce confusion in the public mind about advanced practice nursing. As one NP recently noted, however, "It is possible for this combined role NP to be spread too thinly in trying to execute all of the functions of a greatly expanded role" (Breuninger, 1996, p. 14). The difficulty of one advanced practice nurse performing every service for each client was a compelling reason for the development of a collaborative partnership between the APNs described in the partnership example at the end of the chapter.

Model of Collaborative Practice Between APNs

Although APNs have collaborated with other health professionals since the inception of their practice, most of the literature on collaboration has focused on nurse-physician interaction, or on master's-prepared to baccalaureate nurse interactions. Little can be found about APNs collaborating with one another to manage a shared caseload of clients. Collaboration requires a clear explication of APN roles to gain a clear idea of where roles differentiate and where they overlap. Changes in role functions and practice settings make this differentiation essential for all advanced practice nurses.

Differentiation of the nurse case manager role is in its infancy, so a discussion of advanced practice nurses must compare the "second generation"

CNS and the FNP. A number of nurses have discussed the differences between clinical nurse specialist and family nurse practitioner roles. Hanson and Martin (1990) discussed NP and CNS functions. In their view, the NP emphasizes health promotion and illness prevention in community-based settings; the CNS works with tertiary health concerns in a hospital-based practice.

These distinctions, however, are becoming blurred as managed care changes the health care environment. Nurse practitioners are taking on more hospital-based care; clinical nurse specialists (functioning as NCMs) are following chronically ill people into community-based settings (Cronenwett, 1995; Hanson, 1991). Delineating the difference between APN roles allows for partnerships that use the strengths of the specific type of advanced practice.

Specific Functions

Figure 15.1 is a model of the separate and shared functions of family nurse practitioners and NCMs in a primary care setting. Family nurse practitioners emphasize health promotion and disease prevention within a context of family-focused primary care (Hanson & Martin, 1990). Unique functions of FNPs are assessment, diagnosis, and management of primary care health concerns, using both medical and nursing models. FNPs also order and monitor medical therapies.

Nurse case managers aid clients to achieve maximum self-care capabilities (Conger, 1996). To do so, they assess, diagnose, and manage client and environmental systems; provide extended client education and counseling; assist clients to navigate the healthcare system; and coordinate care (Conger, 1996). In direct client care, they become a "cheerleader" for the client.

In a partnership between an NCM and a family nurse practitioner, some departure from "traditional" roles may be required. The NCM will have a greater emphasis on direct client care; the FNP will do less patient education and counseling. Client outcomes of quality care through enhanced self-care abilities and cost-effective care through health promotion and disease prevention reflect the goals of both advanced practice specialties.

The FNP and NCM share the responsibilities for short-term client and family education and counseling. Both APNs monitor and evaluate the

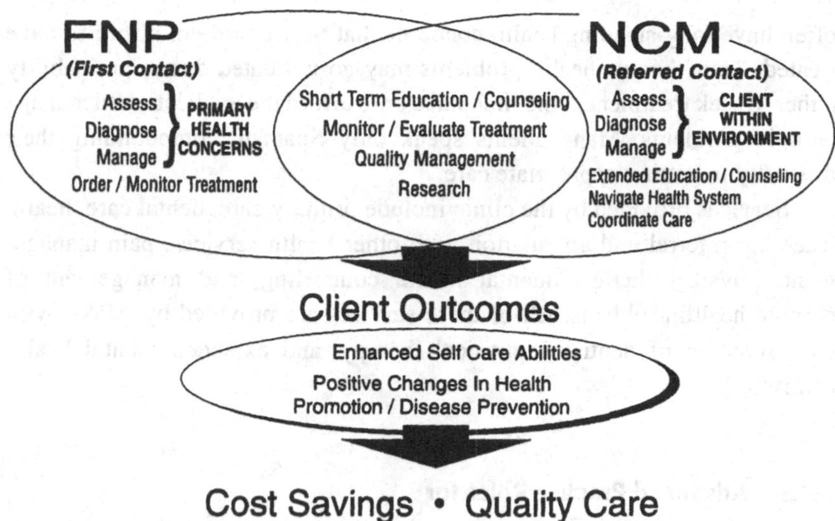

Figure 15.1 Model for Advanced Practice Nurse Collaboration

efficacy of treatments while providing tracking and follow-up of treatment. Quality improvement and research activities also remain a shared responsibility.

Example From Clinical Practice

A search of the nursing literature revealed no discussion of an FNP-NCM collaborative practice and, indeed, very little about APNs working together in any fashion. Therefore, the following discussion is an illustration of our partnership as an FNP and an NCM who share a client caseload.

Center Description

The practice base is in a community health center in rural Northern Arizona. Our clients are primarily the working poor, who have few resources and little or no discretionary income. We see approximately 500 clients per month who range in age across the lifespan. People who come to the clinic often have long-standing health concerns that they could not afford to have treated. Thus, known health problems may go untreated due to an inability either to seek treatment in the first place or to afford the medication to manage chronic problems. Many clients speak only Spanish, compounding their difficulty in getting appropriate care.

Services provided by the clinic include primary care, dental care, health teaching, referral and articulation with other health services, pain management, physical therapy, mental health counseling, and management of chronic health problems. All of these services are provided by APNs, with the exception of dentistry, physical therapy, and extended mental health counseling.

Advanced Practice Roles for Nurses in the Center

Family Nurse Practitioner

Our separate activities reflect our specialties in practice and, to some extent, our unique clinical experiences. The FNP is the first contact for all new clients who become part of our shared caseload. An in-depth assessment is made of the client and family, focused around the primary health care concerns. From the assessment, the FNP provides the diagnosis and management of acute and chronic health concerns in addition to a focus on health promotion and disease prevention activities. Arizona FNPs have prescriptive authority, so this FNP has the responsibility of prescribing and managing medications as well. The goal of the FNP is to restore health and promote high-level wellness through the client's health promotion and disease prevention activities.

Not everyone who comes to the clinic needs the extensive collaborative services that a partnership between an FNP and a NCM has to offer. The criteria for referral to the case manager are

- multiple physical and/or psychosocial needs
- new onset chronic disorder
- treatment need not provided at center
- client difficulty with management of chronic disorder

Nurse Case Manager

Once the referral is made, the nurse case manager does an extensive assessment of the client's environmental and social situation, which augments the assessment done by the FNP. The NCM continues the assessment of health promotion and disease prevention concerns that the FNP has discussed with the client and family. This assessment is used to guide teaching and health care system concerns for the client and family, with the goal of promoting maximum self-care capabilities.

The NCM provides in-depth health education in both one-to-one and group sessions. Teaching is more formal and more extensive than that provided by the nurse practitioner. The NCM serves as counselor and coach during education sessions to assist clients with increasing self-care abilities. Clients' and families' progress is monitored, and a referral back to the FNP is made when further assessment and management of primary care concerns is necessary.

In addition, the case manager links people with community resources. Many of our clients have extremely limited resources. The case manager finds providers with sliding scales or providers willing to donate their expertise. Agencies are located that will help to provide services and funding to our clients, and the NCM works closely with people to help them negotiate the agencies' systems and services.

Shared Activities

The family nurse practitioner and the nurse case manager provide health promotion and disease prevention services in their daily encounters with patients. Both advanced practice nurses include health education in their client encounters. Everyone does medication teaching as well. The FNPs include information about the medications they have prescribed to the client, and the case manager does in-depth evaluation of medication management by the client and appropriate teaching.

Finally, the APNs are involved in quality management issues in formal and informal ways. The FNP sits on the quality management committee, but both are involved in setting standards and the evaluation of those standards. Research projects are common to both nurses.

Communication Between the APNs

Clients are seen initially by the family nurse practitioner, who determines the need for collaboration with the nurse case manager. The FNP makes a referral, usually verbally, or by leaving a message in the communication boxes. We are both faculty at Northern Arizona University and can discuss client referrals with each other in our offices at the university as well. As clients are seen in collaboration, discussion of their management takes place in formal, weekly conferences and in "corridor conferences" where we discuss progress and problems in an informal way. The collaboration decisions in the formal conferences are charted, and the plan that develops out of more informal collaboration is documented in the chart as well.

Uniqueness of APN Collaboration

Part of what makes this collaboration work well is that nurses prepared at the master's level share a philosophy about people and health care, have common goals, and are comfortable working within a theoretical framework for practice. The following philosophy and goals were established by our work together with clients; it has proven very useful.

Philosophy

Health is defined broadly to include environmental and social influences on both health status and the choices people make about their health care. Close attention is paid, therefore, to income, social status, and cultural factors. When people are seen as holistic beings in an environmental and social context, advanced practice nurses are comfortable with issues as broad-ranging as spiritual concerns and pets as social support. In addition, we believe that people have the right and the responsibility to make their own health care decisions, so time is spent to make certain that people have all of the information they need to make informed choices.

Goals

Our basic goal in collaborative practice is to work with people so that they can manage their health care concerns as independently of the health care system as possible. Conscious effort is made to empower people to have the resources and knowledge to be their own health care providers, with minimal assistance. Teaching and assistance are therefore focused in this direction.

Theoretical Framework

A framework of self-efficacy is used as a guiding principle. As people gain self-efficacy, they are empowered to take control of their health care concerns. This scale is based on social cognitive theory (Bandura, 1986), in which the belief that one has the ability to perform a task influences the degree of effort put into task accomplishment. Another study (Stewart, Keleman, & Ewart, 1994) suggests that positive reinforcement given to a person learning a new behavior can increase that person's self-efficacy. As self-efficacy is increased, self-management behaviors should increase. Master's preparation in nursing gives us a comfort level with the use of theory in clinical practice and provides a guide for interventions.

Factors That Enhance Collaboration

Because APNs have the same preparation, there is no hierarchy in our work together, as there often is between nurses and other professionals. No one "owns" the clients in the clinic; in fact, we believe that the clients own themselves, and we are team members who work together in a problem-solving mode. Therefore, no one needs permission to provide any aspect of care; instead, we work, with the client, towards a mutually acceptable plan. Our team meetings stress collaboration and consensus.

Our educational preparation also gives us an appreciation for one another's special expertise within the profession of nursing. We share a common core of knowledge and beliefs, with an understanding of when collaboration will be most useful.

Evaluation Methodologies

The evaluation of our clients is part of a pilot research project to explore possible measurement of client outcomes in our practice. Evaluation reflects the two outcome goals for our clients: changes in health promotion and disease prevention behaviors and changes in self-care management. These goals in turn provide cost savings, which are measured directly, and quality care, which is measured by positive changes in physiologic and self-efficacy measures. The client knowledge base is continually assessed on an informal basis. Physical parameters that we measure, as appropriate, are body mass index, blood pressure and blood glucose, and relevant laboratory values such as hemoglobin A1c, cholesterol, and lipid values.

Changes in self-care management are measured in part by looking at changes in self-efficacy. For those clients who are working on weight management, the Weight Self-efficacy Scale is administered at the beginning of intervention and again 12 weeks later.

Finally, and very important, we are doing cost-benefit analyses to demonstrate cost savings associated with our collaboration. The theory behind cost benefit analysis arises from case management literature (Mullahy, 1995). The analysis consists both of a calculation of what the present level of services to provide care for a client is costing and a projected calculation of services avoided by effective case management. Cost of services includes provider services, supply charges, and institutional charges. This type of analysis is especially important as we move into aggressive health promotion activities because the outcome of such activity cannot be measured in more traditional ways.

To perform a cost analysis, one first calculates the cost of the present level of service, then the cost of potential services that would be required if case management had not occurred. Finally, the net savings due to case management are determined. Net savings are determined by subtracting actual costs from potential savings.

The potential savings are calculated as both hard and soft savings. Hard savings include such things as the difference in cost between caring for a client in an acute-care facility as opposed to skilled nursing. The soft savings are more difficult to compute but are vital to demonstrating nursing effectiveness. These would include savings obtained by avoiding an inpatient hospitalization or reduced morbidity because of the case management activities.

Client Situations

Our methods can perhaps best be illustrated through the use of two case studies. A typical client with long-term health issues, a 55-year-old woman, first came to the center in a wheelchair, unable to walk because of both back and knee pain. She had diabetes mellitus, and her blood sugars were in the 300 mg range. Her last physician had given up, saying that she would always have uncontrolled diabetes. Her vision was so blurred that she was unable to read her Bible, which was a source of great distress to her. She worked with the nurse case manager to increase her understanding of diabetes, which was quite limited and contributed to her management difficulties. The family nurse practitioner adjusted her insulin levels and referred her to physical therapy for her back and knee pain. Today she walks without assistive devices, her blood sugars are in the 150 range, her insulin need has been reduced, and she has lost 22 lb. She can once again read her Bible, and she attributes her improved condition to the center and to God.

During our work with this woman, numerous interactions between the APNs occurred. At one point during a case management visit, our client informed us that she had stepped on a rusty nail during the previous week. The only self-care that she had done was to clean the wound. The NCM immediately referred her to the FNP to obtain tetanus toxoid and an evaluation of the wound site. During the next 6 weeks, numerous consultations between APNs took place to help this woman manage her multiple concerns. The FNP took charge of the medication plan; the NCM provided instruction on wound care, advocated for the client to secure a sturdy pair of shoes, arranged for consultation with a podiatrist, and assisted the client in developing an attenuated exercise program during the time she was unable to do her walking program.

A second case situation that demonstrates complex health and social issues was that of a woman who came to the clinic with a diagnosis of chronic fatigue/chronic pain syndrome. She was taking numerous pain medications, including both NSAIDS and narcotics, an antianxiety agent, and an antidepressant, without relief of pain or anxiety. She was seen first by the FNP to review her medications and a tooth infection, then referred to the case manager for assistance in coping with her life. She had recently moved to our community, was not working, had left her only child with her ex-husband, and was very unhappy about a 20-lb weight gain. In her previous community, she had "stayed in bed all day, every day, unable to move."

The NCM worked with her to identify community resources and referred her to the state vocational rehabilitation program for possible work retraining. She was referred to a mental health counselor for management of her depression and anxiety, and the FNP requested special consultation from a psychiatrist for management of her psychiatric medications. The NCM worked with the client to apply for health care assistance.

It was determined after a great deal of consultation that this client would need to stop her narcotics, reduce her reliance on medications for pain management, and work towards more control over her life circumstances. To do this, she was referred to an FNP with experience in nonpharmacologic pain control and to the counselor for depression and anxiety. The NCM assisted with lifestyle adaptations, and the FNP managed general health concerns, such as her infected tooth.

Cost benefits can be calculated with these two clients. The first client was managed by providing tetanus toxoid, wound management, referral to a podiatrist, and getting her a new, more sturdy pair of shoes. This management avoided two possible scenarios: The first scenario was that a hospitalization with tetanus was avoided. If one considers that an episode of tetanus could have resulted in numerous days of hospitalization in an intensive care unit at thousands of dollars per day, the cost of the health management becomes insignificant. Aggressive management of the foot injury also prevented spread of the infection, possibly leading to the need for hospitalization or even amputation with all of its attendant costs. In either of these possible scenarios, the cost of acute-care hospitalization would have run to thousands of dollars.

With the second patient cited, the management of the client led to more subtle cost savings. Reducing her need for narcotic management was fairly insignificant in terms of dollars. However, the case management went beyond merely reducing her need for narcotics. The focus on assisting her with social issues is where possible cost benefits occurred. By assisting her to take control of her life, working with her to develop new vocational skills, and allaying her anxieties so that she could become a more productive member of the community, cost benefits in terms of social programs were realized. The goal for this client is to return her to gainful employment so that she will not be dependent on welfare.

Conclusions

Our collaboration differs from the collaboration between APNs and physicians. Most APN-physician collaboration is that of the nurse referring to the physician; rarely do physicians refer their clients to nurses for care. As APNs, however, we share the care of clients and refer back and forth frequently to one another to maximize client care. We believe that our model of collaboration is important to the development of advanced nursing practice within a managed care environment. The ideas presented in this chapter demonstrate a model of cost-effective care that retains exceptional quality of care for clients. The authors suggest that a managed care organization would do well to consider this model as a means of achieving organization and client objectives.

To achieve the goals of this model, advanced practice nurses will need to be prepared in educational programs in which collaborative practice among nurses is encouraged. This will require rethinking of graduate nurse tracks available to students. Before converting all CNS tracks to nurse practitioner tracks, the benefits derived from collaborative practice among APNs should be considered.

References

Bandura, A. (1986). *Social foundations of thought and action: A social cognitive theory*. Englewood Cliffs, NJ: Prentice Hall.

Breuninger, K. (1996). CNS and NP role merger? *Nurse Practitioner, 21*(11), 12, 14.

Conger, M. (1996). Integration of the clinical nurse specialist into the nurse case manager role. *Nursing Case Management, 1*(5), 230-234.

Cronenwett, L. R. (1995). Molding the future of advanced practice nursing. *Nursing Outlook, 43*(3), 112-118.

Elder, R. G., & Bullough, B. (1990). Practitioners and clinical nurse specialists: Are the roles merging? *Clinical Nurse Specialist, 4*(2), 78-84.

Haddock, K. S. (1997). Clinical nurse specialist. In S. Moorhead & D. Huber (Eds.), *Nursing roles: Evolving or recycled*? (pp. 139-149). Thousand Oaks, CA: Sage.

Hanson, C. M. (1991). The 1990's and beyond: Determining the need for community health and primary care nurses for rural populations. *Journal of Rural Health, 7*(1), 413-426.

Hanson, C. M., & Martin, L. L. (1990). The nurse practitioner and clinical nurse specialist: Should the roles be merged? *Journal of the American Academy of Nurse Practitioners*, *2*(1), 2-9.

Jenkins, M. L., & Sullivan-Marx, E. M. (1994). Nurse practitioners and community health nurses: Clinical partnerships and future visions. *Nursing Clinics of North America*, *29*(3), 459-470.

Mullahy, C. M. (1995). *The case manager's handbook*. Gaithersburg, MD: Aspen.

Pender, N. J. (1992). Partnerships: An alternative to rugged individualism. *Nursing Outlook*, *40*(6), 248-249.

Schroer, K. (1991). Case management: Clinical nurse specialist and nurse practitioner, converging roles. *Clinical Nurse Specialist*, *8*(4), 189-194.

Stewart, K., Keleman, M. H., & Ewart, C. K. (1994). Relationships between self-efficacy and mood before and after exercise training. *Journal of Cardiopulmonary Rehabilitation*, *14*, 35-42.

Walker, M. K., & Sebastian, J. G. (1997). Complementarity of advanced practice nursing role in enhancing health outcomes of the chronically ill: Acute care nurse practitioners and nurse case managers. In S. Moorhead & D. G. Huber (Eds.), *Nursing roles: Evolving or recycled?* (pp. 170-190). Thousand Oaks, CA: Sage.

Index

Accreditation, 10-11, 14
Acute-care hospital practice, 111-112
    admission activities, 154-159, 156 (table)
    discharge process, 171-173
    nurse case manager and, 167-170, 173
    patient progress review, 159-167, 164 (figures), 165 (figure)
Acute-care nurse practitioner (ACNP), 142
    clinical nurse specialist and, 147-149
    practice issues, 145-146
    practice settings, 142-144
    reporting issues, 146-147
    standards for practice, 144
Acute-care services, 19-20, 95-96, 101-102
Advanced practice nurses (APN), 4, 103, 105, 135-136, 149-150, 240, 243-244
    case management and, 240-243, 254
    clinical nurse specialist (CNS), 140-142, 239-240
    competencies, applications of, 243-248
    nurse anesthetist (CRNAs), 137-138
    nurse midwife (CNM), 138-140
    primary health care settings and, 270
    seven domains of, 241, 242-243
    worker's compensation-based case management, 248-254, 254 (table)
    See also Collaborative practice; Community health clinics
American Association of Colleges of Nursing, 103, 104
American Association of Retired People (AARP), 6, 10, 11, 231
American Nurses Association (ANA), 68, 77-78, 94
American Nurses Credentialing Center, 104
ANA Safety and Quality Initiative Task Force, 78, 79
Automated clinical pathways. *See* Clinical pathways

Capitation principles, 25-26
Care delivery:
    coordination of care, 51-57
    factors affecting 9-11, 10 (figure)
    See also Cost containment; Nurse extenders; Quality of care
Case management. *See* Community-based care; Nurse case management; Population-based care
Case Management Society of America, 104
Certified nurse midwife (CNM), 138-140
Certified nursing assistant (CNA), 116-120
Certified registered nurse anesthetist (CRNA), 137-138
Chronic conditions, 19-20, 57
Clinical nurse specialist (CNS), 103, 135-136, 140-142, 147-149, 271, 272
Clinical pathways, 175-177, 192
    automation, advantages of, 177-179

computerized charting system and, 182-185, 183-184 (figures), 186 (figure), 190-191
interdisciplinary development of, 179-181
legal implications of, 185-190
outcome-focused care, 181-182
permanent record, 177
See also Outcome research
Clinics. *See* Community health clinics
Coalition for Health Care Choice and Accountability, 11
Code for Nurses, 68, 80
Collaborative practice, 269-270
advanced practice nurses, roles of, 271
clinical example of, 273-274
cost benefits, 280-281
evaluation methodologies, 278-281
features of, 276-277
front-line practice roles, 274-276
model of, 271-273, 273 (figure), 281
primary health care settings and, 270
Community-based care, 9, 18, 93-94, 96-97, 207-208, 209-210, 221
home-based programs, 212-215, 214 (table)
long-term care, 210
nursing home setting, 210-212
parish nursing, 215-219
physician office case management, 219-221
See also Advanced practice nurses; Community health clinics
Community health clinics:
advanced practice nurses and, 257-258
teen population, 258-262
uninsured populations, 262-265
Congestive heart failure, 199-202, 200 (table), 245 (table), 247-248
Consolidations/mergers, 18
Consumer Coalition for Quality Health Care, 11
Consumer protection, 19-20
Continuous quality improvement (CQI), 63, 70-72, 71 (figure)
Coordination of care, 51-52
availability of services, 56
choice of provider, 52-53
communication systems, 55
gatekeeper control, 53
hand-off times, 56-57
precertification, 53-54
utilization management, 54-55
Cost containment, 7-10, 8 (table), 10 (figure)
consolidation/merger, 18
for-profit care, 18, 36-37
integration of services, 48-51
outpatient care, 17
peer review, 16-17
private insurers, 17-18
regional planning groups, 15-16
Cost-effectiveness, measurement of, 83-84
cost-benefit analysis, 85-87, 87 (table)
resource utilization, 84-85
Critical pathways. *See* Clinical pathways

Delegation decision making, 124-128, 129 (figure)
Diagnostic Related Groups (DRG), 17
Diagnostic services, 9, 17
Documentation. *See* Clinical pathways
Donabedian assessment model, 68-69

Economic issues, 5-6
cost containment, 7-9, 8 (table), 10 (figure), 15-18
financial risk, 34-36, 35 (figure)
market forces, 9-11, 10 (figure)
post-World War II boom, 12-14, 13 (figure)
Education for the Handicapped Act, 228
Elderly population. *See* Geriatric population
Exclusive provider organization (EPO), 32

Family health care:
elderly, 230-236
infants, special needs, 228-229
pregnancy, high-risk, 230
Family nurse practitioner (FNP), 270, 272, 273 (figure), 274
Federally financed care, 37
Indian Health Service, 42-43
Medicaid HMO, 39-41
Medicare HMO, 37-39
Financial risk, 34-36, 35 (figure)
For-profit care, 18, 36-37

Gag rules, 19
Gatekeeper, 8, 26, 53
Geriatric population, 6, 11, 17, 37-39, 230-231
case management need, 232-233, 234 (table)
community health centers and, 233-235
health care system limitations, 231-232, 232 (table)
limited-functioning patients, 235-236
Great Society era, 12, 13 (figure)
Group Health Cooperative, 25, 27

Health Care Financing Administration (HCFA), 11, 16, 34, 37-38
Health maintenance organizations (HMO), 25, 26-27
federal financing of, 37-41
group model, 28-29
independent practice association (IPA), 30
network model, 29-30
staff model, 27-28, 28 (table)
Health promotion. *See* Wellness promotion
Hill-Burton Act, 13, 18
HIV/AIDS, 245 (table), 246-247
Home health industry, 9, 17, 212-215, 214 (table)
Homeless populations, 226-228
Hospital practice. *See* Acute-care hospital practice

Independent practice associations (IPA), 30
Indian Health Service (IHS), 42-43
Indicators of quality care:
nurse-sensitive, 74-77, 75 (table)
traditional, 74
Information management systems. *See* Clinical pathways
Integration of services, 48-49
clinical integration, 50-51
functional integration, 50
physician system integration, 51

Joint Commission on the Accreditation of Health Care Organizations (JCAHO), 11, 14, 69

Kaiser Foundation Health Plan 25, 29

Laboratory testing, 8, 9
Length of stay (LOS), 74, 196-197, 248
Licensed practical nurse (LPN), 115-119

Malpractice litigation, 185-190, 192
Managed care:
care delivery, 9-11, 10 (figure), 18-19, 51-57
defined, 24-25
nursing role and, 4-6, 20
profit motive, 7, 18, 36-37
See also Economic issues; Organizational structures; Organizations; Practice strategies
Market forces, 9-11, 10 (figure)
Medicaid, 39-41, 226
Medicare, 6, 11, 12-13, 102
cost containment, 16-17
HMO plans and, 37-39
Mental illness, 244-245 (table)
Mergers/consolidations, 18
Migrant workers, 226-228
Morbidity/mortality, 74

National Committee on Quality Assurance (NCOA), 10
National Council of State Boards of Nursing, The, 125-126
National League for Nursing, 82
Need levels, 105-107, 106 (table)
Nonprofit organizations, 36-37
Nurse case management, 57, 91-92, 107, 153-154
acute-care model of, 95-96, 167-170
collaborative practice, 270-275
community-based model of, 96-97
defined, 94
educational preparation for, 102-105
goals of, 97-99, 98 (table)
need criteria, 105-107, 106 (table)
origins of, 92-94
personnel, 101-102
physician office case management, 219-221

skills required for, 99-101, 100 (table)
See also Acute-care hospital practice; Advanced practice nurses; Community-based care; Nurse extenders; Population-based care
Nurse case manager (NCM). *See* Nurse case management
Nurse extenders, 113-114, 115-116, 132
delegation of duties and, 126-127
educational programs for, 119-120
reasons for use, 114-115
registered nurses and, 120-123, 122 (table)
regulation of, 116-117, 126-127
use of currently, 117-119, 119 (table)
Nursing:
care evaluation, 74-77, 75 (table), 81 (figure), 82-83
communication skills, 124
delegation decision making, 124-128, 129 (figure)
ethical principles in, 80-82, 81 (figure)
managed care and, 20
process strategies, 128-129
reorganization of, 4-5, 6
teamwork in, 123-132, 129 (figure), 131 (figure)
threats to, 5-6
unlicensed personnel/RN, roles of, 120-123, 122 (table)
utilization management and, 54-55
See also Advanced practice nurses; Nurse case management; Patient care evaluation; Quality of care
Nursing home care, 210-212
Nursing Interventions Classification (NIC), 265, 266 (table)

Organizational structures, 23-24
alternative, 30-34, 31 (table)
capitation principles, 25-26
financial risk, 34-36, 35 (figure)
for-profit/not-for-profit, 36-37
health maintenance organizations, 26-30, 28 (table)
managed care defined, 24-25
See also Nurse case management
Organizations, 6-7
characteristics of, 7-9, 8 (table)
focus of, 18-19
Outcome management, 72-73, 73 (table), 78-79, 81 figure), 82-83
Outcome research, 195-196, 204-205
congestive heart failure, study results, 199-202, 200 table)
outcome studies, 196-197
study design, 197-199
total hip replacement, study results, 202-204, 203 (table)
Outpatient care, 17

Parish nursing, 215-219
Patient care evaluation, 68-69
collaborative practice, 278-281
continuous quality improvement (CQI), 70-72, 71 (figure)
outcome management, 72-73, 73 (table), 78-79
quality assurance methodologies, 69
total quality management (TQM), 70
Patient progress review, 159-167, 164 (figures), 165 (figure)
Patient record. *See* Clinical pathways
Patient service associate (PSA), 118
Peer review, 16-17
Peer Review Organization (PRO), 16, 101
Physician-hospital organization (PHO), 32
Physician network, 33-34
Point-of-service plan, 53
Population-based care, 223-224, 236-237, 254-255
development of, 224-226
elderly, 230-236
infants, special needs, 228-229
living circumstances and, 226-228
pregnancy, high-risk, 230
Practice strategies, 47-48
coordination of care, 51-57
integration of services, 48-51
quality management, 61-64
wellness promotion, 57-61
See also Nurse case management; Nurse extenders
Preexisting conditions, 19
Preferred provider organization (PPO), 31-32

Presidential Advisory Commission on Consumer Protection and Quality, 10
Private insurance plans, 17-18
Professional Standards Review Organization (PSRO), 16
Profit motivation, 7
Progress review. *See* Patient progress review
Public health, 58-60, 93

Quality management, 61, 63-64
  defined, 61-62
  programs, 62-63
Quality of care, 67-68, 87-88
  cost benefit analysis, 85-87, 87 (table)
  cost effectiveness and, 83-84
  indicators of, 74-80
  measurement techniques, 68-73, 71 (figure), 73 (table)
  outcome measurement, 78-79, 81 (figure), 82-83
  resource utilization, 79-80, 84-85
  risk management, 77-78
Quality review, 10-11

Research. *See* Outcome research
Resources:
  allocation, 83-84
  utilization, 79-80, 81, 84-85
  See also Outcome research

School-linked clinics, 259, 260-262
Screening tools, 105, 106 (table), 107
Social capital, 18
Social morbidity, 258-259
Social Security Act, 12-13
Strategies. *See* Practice strategies

Team nursing, 122-123
  case study, 129-132, 131 (figure)
  clinical pathways and, 176-177
  communication skills, 124
  delegation decision making, 124-128, 129 (figure)
  process strategies, 128-129
  See also Collaborative practice
Technology, 14, 83-84
Teen population, 258-262
Testing. *See* Laboratory testing
Total quality management (TQM), 62-63, 70

United States:
  cost containment, 15-18, 15 (figure)
  federally financed care, 37-43
  health care expansion, 12-14, 13 (figure)
Unlicensed assistive personnel (UAP), 118-119, 119 (table)
Utilization management, 54-55
Utilization review nurse (URN), 101-102

Variance analysis, 161-162, 166-167, 182

Wellness promotion, xii, 8-9, 18
  education, 60-61
  parish nursing, 215-219
  prenatal care, 60
  preventive care cost, 57-58
  public health and, 58-60
Worker's compensation-based case management, 248-250
  absence of management, 250-252
  cost comparison, 253-254, 254 (table)
  utilization of management, 252-253

Zander case management model, 96

About the Editor

Margaret M. Conger, RN, EdD, is Associate Professor of Nursing at Northern Arizona University. Her teaching responsibilities there focus on the development of a rural health clinical track in the graduate program that includes a strong focus on case management principles as applied in the managed care environment. She has completed postgraduate work in case management at the University of Arizona and has a number of publications in this area.

About the Contributors

Lisa Brugh, RN, MS OCN, is the Clinical Pathways Coordinator at Flagstaff Medical Center in Flagstaff, Arizona, where she has facilitated the development of over 20 automated clinical pathways. She has done graduate work at Northern Arizona University, where her emphasis is on case management strategies that enhance collaborative care practices.

Carol E. Craig, RN, PhD FNPc, is Associate Professor in Nursing at the Oregon Health Sciences Center at Oregon Institute of Technology. She was formerly an Associate Professor of Nursing at Northern Arizona University. She is a certified Family Nurse Practitioner and has maintained her practice at the North Country Community Health Center. She was instrumental in establishing this center as a free clinic to serve the needs of the medically underserved in the community, and she obtained federal funding for the project.

Teri Fernandez, RN, MS, is the owner of Northland Medical Case Management in Prescott, Arizona, where she actively works as a case manager with worker's compensation clients. She has had extensive experience in community-based case management services. She has also participated in developing items for case management certification exams.

Kathy Ingleses, RN, MS, FNP, is Assistant Clinical Professor in Nursing at Northern Arizona University. She also practices as a Family Nurse Practitioner at The Teen Clinic, which is a part of the School-based, School-linked Services program through the Coconino Department of Health Services in Flagstaff, Arizona.

Pamela Keberlein, RN, MSN, is the nursing coordinator for the bedside computer system at Flagstaff Medical Center, Flagstaff, Arizona. In this role, she developed and implemented one of the first bedside computer systems in the United States that incorporated the clinical pathway as part of the documentation system. She has had many years of clinical nursing experience in critical care and surgery. Her current research interests are the effects of managed care and clinical pathways on patient care.

Deanne Lewis, RN, MS, is actively working in case management with worker's compensation clients and is also teaching case management to nursing students. She has had extensive experience in community health nursing.

JoAnne Woodall, RN, MSN, is currently the team leader for case management at Tucson Medical Center in Tucson, Arizona. She developed the first case management program at Flagstaff Medical Center and has done postgraduate work in case management at the University of Arizona.

Printed in the United States
By Bookmasters

Printed in the United States
By Bookmasters